Physiology for General Surgical Sciences
Examination (GSSE)

S. Ali Mirjalili
Editor

Physiology for General Surgical Sciences Examination (GSSE)

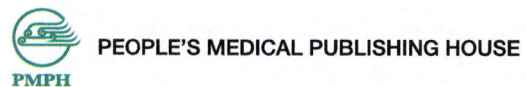 PEOPLE'S MEDICAL PUBLISHING HOUSE 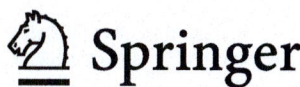 Springer

Editor
S. Ali Mirjalili
Department of Anatomy and Medical Imaging
University of Auckland
Auckland, New Zealand

ISBN 978-981-13-2579-3   ISBN 978-981-13-2580-9 (eBook)
https://doi.org/10.1007/978-981-13-2580-9

© Springer Nature Singapore Pte Ltd. and People's Medical Publishing House Co. Ltd. 2019
This work is subject to copyright. All rights are reserved by the Publisher, whether the whole or part of the material is concerned, specifically the rights of translation, reprinting, reuse of illustrations, recitation, broadcasting, reproduction on microfilms or in any other physical way, and transmission or information storage and retrieval, electronic adaptation, computer software, or by similar or dissimilar methodology now known or hereafter developed.
The use of general descriptive names, registered names, trademarks, service marks, etc. in this publication does not imply, even in the absence of a specific statement, that such names are exempt from the relevant protective laws and regulations and therefore free for general use.
The publisher, the authors, and the editors are safe to assume that the advice and information in this book are believed to be true and accurate at the date of publication. Neither the publisher nor the authors or the editors give a warranty, express or implied, with respect to the material contained herein or for any errors or omissions that may have been made. The publisher remains neutral with regard to jurisdictional claims in published maps and institutional affiliations.

This Springer imprint is published by the registered company Springer Nature Singapore Pte Ltd.
The registered company address is: 152 Beach Road, #21-01/04 Gateway East, Singapore 189721, Singapore

Contents

1 **Endocrine and Reproductive Physiology** 1
   S. Ali Mirjalili, Lucy Hinton, and Simon Richards

2 **Gastrointestinal Physiology** 37
   S. Ali Mirjalili, Lucy Hinton, and Simon Richards

3 **Cardiovascular Physiology** 55
   S. Ali Mirjalili, Lucy Hinton, and Kevin Ellyett

4 **Respiratory Physiology** 89
   S. Ali Mirjalili, Lucy Hinton, and Kevin Ellyett

5 **Renal Physiology** 117
   S. Ali Mirjalili, Lucy Hinton, and Kevin Ellyett

Index.. 139

Chapter 1
Endocrine and Reproductive Physiology

S. Ali Mirjalili, Lucy Hinton, and Simon Richards

1.1 Mechanisms of Hormonal Action

Short notes
Three main types of hormones:

1. Steroid (Lipid soluble): Synthesised from cholesterol. Diffuse out of cell through phospholipid bi-layer. Need to be bound to plasma proteins.
2. Peptide/Protein (Water soluble): Usually formed from a precursor, which is cleaved prior to leaving the cell. Stored in cytoplasmic granules. Released by exocytosis.
3. Amino acid tyrosine derivatives (Water soluble): Thyroid and adrenal medulla hormones.

Function of hormones:
Hormones may act at the cell surface or diffuse into the cell to act on nuclear receptors:

Hormones may act by entering the cell surface → cytoplasmic/nuclear receptors → modify mRNAs

- e.g. thyroid hormones, steroid hormones, vitamin D
    - Steroid hormones can diffuse (or be transported) through the cell membrane
    - Binding may occur in the cytoplasm or nuclear membrane
    - Receptor may then bind to specific parts of the DNA (serum response element or SRE) and regulate mRNA transcription

Hormones may function by acting at the cell surface

- By altering ion movements (often regarded as neurotransmitters) and binding directly to ion channels
    - e.g. $Na^+ - K^+$, GABA/glycine – Cl^-, Nicotinic Acetylcholine receptor

- By ↑ or ↓ adenylate cyclase → ↑ or ↓ production of cyclic AMP (cAMP), by converting ATP to cAMP via G-proteins. cAMP binds to the regulatory subunit of a specific protein kinase
    - e.g. PTH, TSH, Glucagon, ACTH, Catecholamines via beta-1 receptors → ↑ cAMP
    - Catecholamines acting via alpha-2 → ↓ cAMP

- By ↑ guanylate cyclase → ↑ cGMP → e.g. ANP and NO. Similar process as above. Initial action may span the cell membrane [with intra and extracellular functions (ANP)], or act entirely intracellularly (NO)]
- By activating phospholipase C → hydrolysis of cell membrane phospholipids → IP3 and diacylglycerol
    - IP3 → binds to ER → Ca^{2+} release (3rd messenger)
    - Diacylglycerol → ↑ protein kinase C → phosphorylates proteins and alters their function
    - e.g. vasopressin, TRH, angiotensin II, catecholamines via alpha receptors

- By acting on tyrosine kinase → ↑ activity
    - Occurs by spanning membrane → activates tyrosine kinase
    - e.g. insulin, EGF, PDGF

- By linking to intracellular tyrosine kinase
    - e.g. cytokines, GH

1   Endocrine and Reproductive Physiology

1.2   Hypothalamus and Posterior Pituitary

Questions

1. How is thirst controlled by the hypothalamus?

    - By sensing changes in plasma osmolarity through osmoreceptors (anterior hypothalamus)
    - By sensing blood volume changes through angiotensin II
    - By sensing blood volume changes through baroreceptors peripherally

2. Explain the control mechanism for release of hormones from the posterior pituitary.
   Posterior pituitary hormones are synthesised by cell bodies in the hypothalamus. These cells are known as magnocellular neurons in the supraoptic and paraventricular nuclei of the hypothalamus. The pathway from the hypothalamus to the posterior pituitary is called the hypothalamo-neurohypophyseal tract. The hormones (ADH and oxytocin) are stored in vesicles, which are released following various neural stimuli.

3. Explain the mechanism of action of ADH.
   Its main action is to prevent the loss of water in the kidneys by concentrating urine.

    - Acts on renal collecting ducts to ↑ permeability to water passing from urine to medullary fluid (via V2 → cAMP → ↑ water channels from endosomes)
    - Secondary actions are;
    - Increases urea permeability in the collecting ducts of the inner medulla of the kidney
    - Vasoconstriction via V1a → G-protein → ↑ in Ca^{2+} → blood vessel constriction
        - Seen in liver, brain, kidney, mesangial cells
    - Stimulation of ACTH release by corticotrophins in the anterior pituitary via V1b → G-protein → Ca^{2+} release
    - Stimulation of glycogen breakdown in the liver

4. What are the effects of oxytocin?

    - Contraction of myoepithelial cells in the breast → milk ejection
    - Contraction of smooth muscle of uterus
    - ADH effect in high concentrations

5. What is diabetes insipidus?
   This is a condition where the body has an abnormal inability to secrete or respond to ADH. May be due to destruction (neoplasm/trauma) of hypothalamus (neurogenic) leading to lack of ADH, or due to inability of the kidney (nephrogenic) to

respond to ADH (acquired or genetic). It results in water loss through the kidneys resulting in polydipsia, polyuria (often >20 L/day) and thirst.

<u>Short notes</u>
Functions of the hypothalamus

1. Control of anterior pituitary hormone secretion (via releasing hormones) <u>*see text of anterior pituitary*</u>.
2. Control of appetite
   - Lateral feeding centre chronically active but suppressed by satiety centre and possibly CCK and leptin
   - Ventrolateral satiety centre senses glucose utilisation and is insulin sensitive
3. Role in cyclic phenomena - circadian rhythms, body temperature
4. Control of thirst
   - By sensing changes in plasma osmolarity through osmoreceptors (anterior hypothalamus)
   - By sensing blood volume changes through angiotensin II
   - By sensing blood volume changes through baroreceptors peripherally → nerves
5. Control of posterior pituitary secretion (vasopressin/ADH, oxytocin)
   - Formed as preprohormones
6. Vasopressin (ADH)
   - Stimulated by anti-diuretic hormone mechanisms
     – ↑ in plasma osmotic pressure (sensed by anterior hypothalamus)
     – ↓ in plasma volume (sensed by baroreceptors – overrides osmotic effect)
     – Angiotensin II
     – Stress and pain
     – Drugs (morphine, nicotine)
     – Sleep
   - Inhibited by pro-diuretic mechanisms
     – ↓ in plasma osmotic pressure
     – ↑ in plasma volume
     – Alcohol
   - Not bound in plasma, readily distributed, degraded by proteolysis
   - Actions
     - Antidiuretic action
       – Acts on collecting ducts to ↑ permeability to water passing from urine to medullary fluid (via V2 receptor→ cAMP → ↑ water channels from endosomes)
       – Increases urea permeability in the collecting ducts of the inner medulla of the kidney

1 Endocrine and Reproductive Physiology

- Vasoconstriction
  - Via V1a receptor → G-protein → ↑ in Ca^{2+} → blood vessel constriction
  - Seen in liver, brain, kidney, mesangial cells
- Stimulation of ACTH release by corticotrophins in the anterior pituitary via V1b receptor → G-protein → Ca^{2+} release
- Stimulation of glycogen breakdown in the liver
- Diabetes insipidus
  - May result from destruction (neoplasm / trauma) of hypothalamus (neurogenic) leading to a lack of ADH, or due to inability of the kidney (nephrogenic) to respond to ADH (acquired or genetic)

7. Oxytocin (hormone related to ADH)
   - Stimulated by mechanical vaginal distension, nipple stimulation, stress
   - Inhibited by Alcohol
   - Actions:
     - Contraction of myoepithelial cells in the breast → milk ejection
     - Contraction of smooth muscle of uterus
     - ADH effect in high concentrations
   - Effects mediated by specific receptor → G protein → Ca^{2+} release
   - Number of receptors increases dramatically during late stages of pregnancy

8. Pineal gland
   - Secretes melatonin cyclically (high at night, low during the day)

1.3 Anterior Pituitary

Questions

1. Which cells of the anterior pituitary release TSH, LH, FSH, ACTH, GH and Prolactin?

Hormone	Cell type
TSH	Thyrotrophs
LH	Gonadotrophs
FSH	Gonadotrophs
ACTH	Corticotrophs
GH	Somatotrophs
Prolactin	Lactotrophs

2. What stimulates the release of GH?
   Its release occurs when there is a decrease in metabolic fuels [e.g. hypoglycaemia, ketosis] as well as stress, sleep, glucagon, fasting and L-dopa.
3. What is somatostatin?
   This is a hormone, also known as growth hormone–inhibiting hormone (GHIH), which is released by the hypothalamus and inhibits release of GH.
4. What are the direct effects of GH release?
   Think of GH as increasing protein stores, decreasing fat stores and conserving carbohydrates.
   Direct effects of GH include:

   - Carbohydrate: ↓ glucose uptake by cells, stimulates hepatic glucose output and ↑ insulin secretion.
   - Fat: Stimulates lipolysis and mobilisation of fatty acids from adipose tissue, ↑ conversion of fatty acids to acetyl coenzyme A
   - Protein: ↑ amino acid uptake, ↑ RNA translocation, ↓ catabolism of protein and amino acids.
   - Bone: ↑ protein deposition, ↑ cell reproduction, ↑ osteogenic cells
   - Stimulates erythropoiesis

5. What are somatomedins?
   Somatomedins are a group of proteins released from the liver that promote cell growth and division in response to stimulation by growth hormone (GH)

Short notes
Hormones of the Anterior Pituitary

Hormone	Cell type	Releasing hormone	Inhibiting hormone	Type
TSH	Thyrotrophs	TRH	–	Glycoprotein
LH	Gonadotrophs	LHRH	–	Glycoprotein
FSH	Gonadotrophs	GnRH	–	Glycoprotein
ACTH	Corticotrophs	CRH	–	Single pp
GH	Somatotrophs	GHRH	Somatostatin	Single pp
Prolactin	Lactotrophs	–	Dopamine	Single pp

Release is regulated by the hypothalamus
Glycoproteins are composed of an α subunit (identical) and β subunit (differs)
Please see texts for details on TSH, LH and FSH, ACTH

Growth Hormone (GH)
Does not act on a specific organ but exerts its effect directly on almost all tissues of the body.

- Related structurally to prolactin
- Circulates bound to carrier proteins with a t ½ of 20 min
- Secretion is pulsatile
- Presence of fuels inhibits secretion and vice versa

1 Endocrine and Reproductive Physiology

- ↑ by GHRH (Growth hormone releasing hormone) in response to
  ↓ in metabolic fuels (e.g. ketosis, hypoglycaemia), certain amino acids, stress, deep sleep, sex steroids, glucagon, exercise, fasting, ghrelin, and L-dopa.
- ↓ by GHIH (Growth hormone inhibitory hormone/somatostatin) in response to
  Free fatty acids, glucose
- IGF-I (insulin-like growth factor-I) provides negative feedback

- Stimulates IGF-I production by the liver

  Think of GH as increasing protein deposition, decreasing fat stores and conserving carbohydrates.

- Direct effects of GH include
  - Carbohydrate: ↓ glucose uptake by cells, stimulates hepatic glucose output and ↑ insulin secretion.
  - Fat: Stimulates lipolysis and mobilisation of fatty acids from adipose tissue, ↑ conversion of fatty acids to acetyl coenzyme A
  - Protein: ↑ amino acid uptake, ↑ RNA translocation, ↓ catabolism of protein and amino acids.
  - Bone: ↑ protein deposition, ↑ cell reproduction, ↑ osteogenic cells
  - Stimulates erythropoiesis
- Indirect effects are mediated through IGF-I (somatomedins) from the liver.
  - Receptor is large and stimulates intracellular kinases
  - Insulin like effects, glucose uptake, anti-lipolysis etc
- Other family members include EGF, NGF, PDGF
  - Type I receptors bind IGF-I > IGF-II
  - Type II receptors bind IGF II > IGF I
  - Insulin receptors bind insulin > IGF I

Prolactin

- Secreted by lactotrophs, usually under chronic inhibition via dopamine
- Secretion ↑ by
  - Nipple stimulation, stress, pregnancy, hypoglycaemia, oestrogens, exercise
- Secretion ↓ by
  - L-dopa, bromocriptine
- Under normal negative feedback loops, t ½ of 20 min
- Promotes milk <u>secretion</u> by the breasts
- High concentrations of prolactin inhibit LH and FSH action on the gonads and can cause infertility

1.4 Adrenal Medulla

Questions

1. What are catecholamines derived from?
   The amino acid tyrosine (Fig. 1.1).

2. Where is PNMT (phenylethanolamine-N-methyltransferase) found?
   This is the enzyme that converts noradrenaline to adrenaline. It is found in the adrenal medulla and the brain.

3. What hormone is secreted in the largest quantity from the adrenal medulla?
   Adrenaline. Converted from noradrenaline by the enzyme PNMT (phenylethanolamine-N-methyltransferase). Chromaffin cells secrete primarily adrenaline (85%), noradrenaline (15%) and dopamine (small amounts)

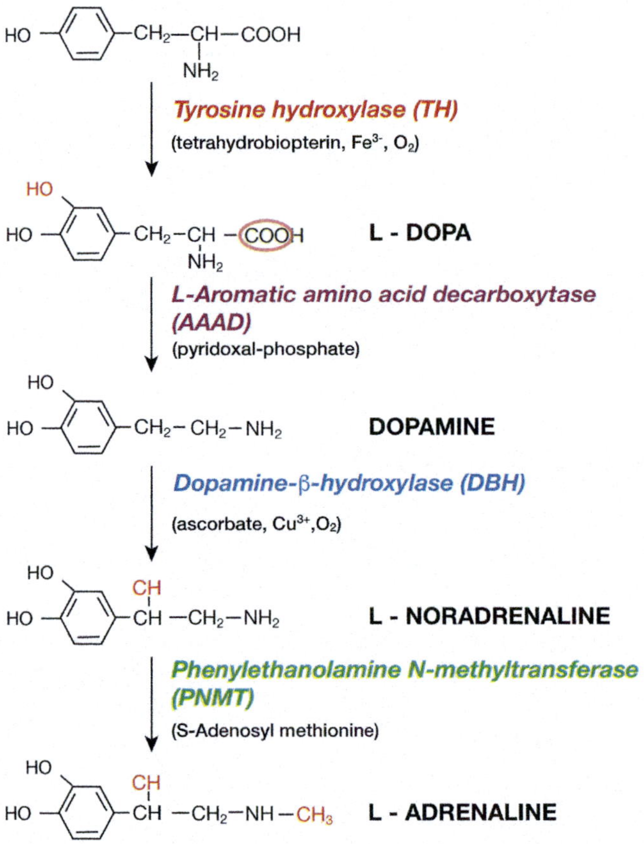

HO—⟨⟩—CH$_2$—CH(NH$_2$)—COOH

↓ **Tyrosine hydroxylase (TH)**
(tetrahydrobiopterin, Fe^{3-}, O$_2$)

HO, HO—⟨⟩—CH$_2$—CH(NH$_2$)—COOH   **L - DOPA**

↓ **L-Aromatic amino acid decarboxylase (AAAD)**
(pyridoxal-phosphate)

HO, HO—⟨⟩—CH$_2$—CH$_2$—NH$_2$ **DOPAMINE**

↓ **Dopamine-β-hydroxylase (DBH)**
(ascorbate, Cu^{3+}, O$_2$)

HO, HO—⟨⟩—CH(OH)—CH$_2$—NH$_2$ **L - NORADRENALINE**

↓ **Phenylethanolamine N-methyltransferase (PNMT)**
(S-Adenosyl methionine)

HO, HO—⟨⟩—CH(OH)—CH$_2$—NH—CH$_3$ **L - ADRENALINE**

Fig. 1.1 Catecholamine production

1 Endocrine and Reproductive Physiology

4. What effect does adrenaline have on the heart?
   It exerts its effects via beta 1 receptors and increases intracellular cAMP. It is an inotrope (↑ contractility) and chronotrope (↑ HR), therefore ↑ SBP and results in a wider pulse pressure.

5. What is a pheochromocytoma?
   This is a rare tumour that secretes catecholamines, either originating in the adrenal medulla or extra-adrenal chromaffin tissue (paraganglioma). It presents with headaches, palpitations and diaphoresis and patients have severe hypertension. Diagnosis is made via measurement of catecholamines and metanephrines in plasma (blood) or 24-h urine collection.

6. How are catecholamines metabolised? Use this to explain the potential harm from the antidepressants, monoamine oxidase inhibitors.
   They can be degraded either by methylation via catechol-O-methyltransferases (COMT) or by deamination via monoamine oxidases (MAO).
   With monoamine oxidase inhibitors, if patients have a diet high in tyramine, excess catecholamines are produced. These cannot be metabolised due to inhibition of the enzyme MAO, leading to excess catecholamines, which can cause a hypertensive crisis.

Short notes
Adrenal Medulla

- Derived from cells from the neural crest (**can be considered a modified sympathetic ganglion**)
- Chromaffin cells are innervated by preganglionic sympathetic fibres and secrete directly into the bloodstream
- Neurotransmitter secreted by the preganglionic axon is acetylcholine

  – Catecholamines synthesised from tyrosine (stored in granules) and dependent on cortisol (t ½ of 2 min)

- Chromaffin cells secrete primarily adrenaline (85%), noradrenaline (15%) and dopamine (small amounts)

  – ↑ secretion by stress, exercise, hypoglycaemia, ↓ secretion by sleep
  – Effects are via adrenergic receptors (α1 and 2, β1 and 2)

	Alpha 1	Alpha 2	Beta 1	Beta 2
Adrenaline	+++	+++	+++	+++
Noradrenaline	+++	+++	+++	+
e.g.	Vasoconstriction Glycogenolysis Intestinal relaxation Pupillary dilation Sweating	Platelet aggregation Vasoconstriction ↓ Insulin secretion	Cardiac stimulation Lipolysis Intestinal relaxation	Bronchodilatation Vasodilation of muscle and liver Uterine relaxation
Mechanism	PLC → IP3 → Ca^{2+}	↓ cAMP	↑ cAMP	↑ cAMP

Release of hormones from adrenal medulla stimulated by:

- 'Stress' – 'fight or flight response'
- Exercise
- Hypoglycaemia

Effects of Adrenaline

- Heart (via β1 "one heart") → ↑ HR, ↑ force, ↑ excitability, ↑ SBP, wider pulse pressure
- Veins (via α1) → vasoconstriction
- Arterioles (α1, α2) → vasoconstriction in most (no effect on cerebral and coronary)
- Skeletal muscle (β2) → vasodilation
- Smooth muscle (β2, α1) → general relaxation, sphincter contraction
- Sweat glands (α1) → ↑ Sweating
- Eye (α1) → pupil dilatation
- Metabolism → ↑ glycogenolysis and lipolysis

Effects of Noradrenaline

- Similar to above but while adrenaline causes vasodilation in skeletal muscle, noradrenaline causes vasoconstriction

Effects of Dopamine

- Acts on α, β1 and β2 and dopaminergic receptors
- Stimulates the heart (via β1), general vasoconstriction but renal vasodilation, ↑ in SBP
- Inhibits prolactin
- Appetite suppressant

Degradation

- Via MAO and secreted in the urine

1.5 Adrenal Cortex

Questions

1. What are the layers of the adrenal cortex and what do they release?
   From out to in; "GFR"
   15% Glomerulosa – Aldosterone (mineralocorticoid)
   75% Fasciculata – Cortisol (glucocorticoids) and androgens
   10% Reticularis – Cortisol (glucocorticoids) and androgens

2. What are adrenal cortex hormones synthesised from?
   Cholesterol (80% of which comes from LDL, some ability to synthesise de novo)

1 Endocrine and Reproductive Physiology

3. What controls secretion of aldosterone?
   Angiotensin II, ACTH, [K$^+$] and [Na$^+$]
   Angiotensin II and K$^+$ are the most important factors.

4. How is cortisol transported in the blood?
   Bound to CBG (corticosteroid-binding globulin/transcortin) (~75%), albumin (~15%) and free (10%).

5. What effects do glucocorticoids have on the body?

   - ↑ protein catabolism
   - ↑ gluconeogenesis
   - anti-insulin effect
   - ↑ blood glucose
   - ↓ glucose utilisation by cells, ↓ GLUT4 in cell membrane
   - ↑ mobilisation and utilisation of fatty acids
   - Anti-inflammatory and immunosuppressive
   - Modulate olfactory stimuli
   - Required for other hormones to work (adrenaline, glucagon, catecholamines → bronchodilatation)
   - Suppresses ACTH secretion (negative feedback)
   - Anti-inflammatory and anti-allergic effects (↓ eosinophils, antibody production and lymphoid organs)
   - ↑ platelets, neutrophils and erythrocytes
   - ↑ HCl and pepsin secretion

6. What are the effects of adrenal insufficiency?
   The term for this is 'Addisons disease' and results in ↓ ECF, hyponatraemia, hyperkalaemia, mild acidosis, hypoglycaemia, ↑ melanin production leading to characteristic pigmentation (due to ACTH stimulation of melanocytes).

7. Explain the pathophysiology of an adrenal crisis.
   This is a medical emergency that can be swiftly fatal if left untreated. It is caused by a deficiency in cortisol and presents with lethargy, hyperkalaemia, hypoglycaemia and hypotension. Treated with hydrocortisone.

   <u>Short notes</u>
   The adrenal cortex has three layers;

1. Glomerulosa (aldosterone)
2. Fasciculata (<u>cortisol</u> and androgens)
3. Reticularis (cortisol and <u>androgens</u>) (Fig. 1.2)

   Mineralocorticoids – Aldosterone

- From zona glomerulosa
- Regulated by

    – ↓ ECF volume → JG cells → renin release → lysis of angiotensinogen → angiotensin I → angiotensin converting-enzyme (lung) → angiotensin II
    – Angiotensin II → stimulates adrenal cortex to produce aldosterone

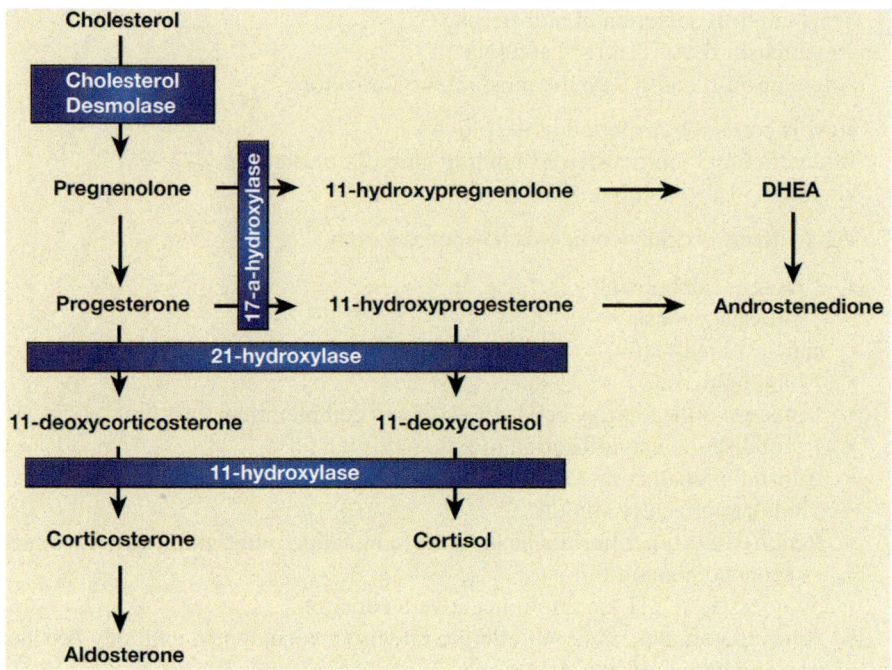

Fig. 1.2 Adrenal cortex hormones

- Hyperkalaemia stimulates aldosterone secretion
- ACTH and Na^+ also have small effects on aldosterone secretion
- Angiotensin II
  - Direct negative feedback and indirect via its actions
  - Powerful vasoconstrictor and ↑ BP
- Production – 0.15 mg/day with concentration of 0.0006 μg/dL.
- Transport and metabolism
  - 60% bound to plasma proteins, 40% free. t ½ of 20 min.
  - Inactivated in the liver by conjugation and reduction – 25% excreted in bile, 75% in urine.
- Effects
  - Lipid soluble, so can be transported through lipid membrane of cells
  - Intracellular aldosterone receptor [mineralocorticoid receptor (MR)] → synthesis of new mRNA → Na^+/K^+ ATP-ase, epithelial sodium channel proteins.
  - Kidney: ↑ distal tubule reabsorption of Na^+ and increases loss of K^+ and H^+

Thus Na⁺ retention and K⁺/H⁺ loss

- Same effect on sweat and salivary glands – increase NaCl resorption and secretion of K^+.
- Large bowel – similar effects

- Excess – In aldosterone excess there is an increase in ECF, however sodium [Na⁺] stays relatively constant. There is hypokalaemia and metabolic alkalosis.
- Deficiency – Severe renal sodium wasting and hyperkalaemia. Total loss causes death in as little as 3 days.

Glucocorticoids

- From zona fasciculata and reticularis, C21, primarily cortisol
- Cortisol synthesised from cholesterol, de novo as required, under control of ACTH
- ACTH
    - CRH (hypothalamus) → corticotrophs → ACTH (AP) → ↑ adenylyl cyclase in the cell membrane to ↑ cAMP → ↑ protein kinase A to change cholesterol to pregnenolone.
    - ↑ by stress (e.g. trauma, infection, surgery) and hypoglycaemia, ↓ by cortisol (negative feedback)
    - Diurnal rhythm (↑ a.m., ↓ at night)

    Trophic action on adrenal cortex
    Melanocyte-stimulating effect (Fig. 1.3)

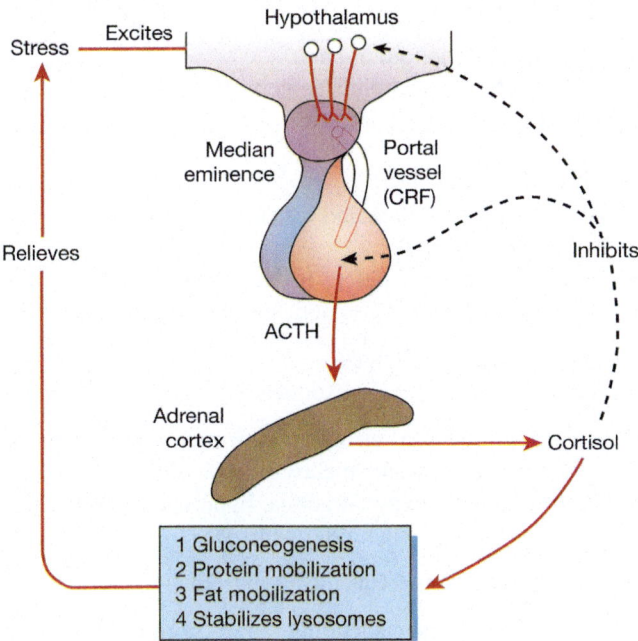

Fig. 1.3 Cortisol release and function

- Production – 10-20 mg/day with a concentration of 12 μg/dL; morning peak.
- Cortisol transport
  - Bound to CBG (corticosteroid-binding globulin/transcortin) (~75%), albumin 11 hydroxylase deficiency → Hypertension, ↑ Na^+ and atypical genitalia
- Metabolism and excretion
  - Mostly converted to cortisone
  - Inactivated in the liver → conjugated → excreted in the kidney
- Action
  - Via receptor to the nucleus → stimulates transcription and ↑ synthesis of mRNA

    ↑ protein catabolism
    ↑ gluconeogenesis
    Anti-insulin effect
    ↑ blood glucose
    ↓ glucose utilisation by cells, ↓ GLUT4 in cell membrane
    ↑ mobilisation and utilisation of fatty acids
    Anti-inflammatory and immunosuppressive
    Modulate olfactory stimuli

  - Required for other hormones to work (adrenaline, glucagon, catecholamines → bronchodilatation)
  - Suppresses ACTH secretion (negative feedback)
  - Anti-inflammatory and anti-allergic effects (↓ eosinophils, antibody production and lymphoid organs)
  - ↑ platelets, neutrophils and erythrocytes
  - ↑ HCl and pepsin secretion

Androgens

- From zona fasciculata and reticularis, most importantly DHEA. Normally only has a weak effect.
- Congenital enzyme defect in the adrenal cortex: 21 hydroxylase deficiency → Na^+ loss; 11 hydroxylase deficiency → Hypertension and ↑ Na^+

Disorders of the adrenals:
Adrenal insufficiency – 'Addison's disease'

- Caused by primary atrophy (80% autoimmune) or injury (TB, Waterhouse–Friderichsen syndrome metastatic disease)
- Effects - ↓ ECF, hyponatraemia, hyperkalaemia and mild acidosis, hypoglycaemia, ↑ melanin production (due to MSH sharing same precursor POMC).

Hyperadrenalism – 'Cushing' syndrome'

- Caused by pituitary adenomas (most common) or ectopic secretion (e.g. paraneoplastic syndrome, adenoma of adrenal cortex).
- Effects – high blood sugar, decreased protein with muscle weakness and osteoporosis, "Cushingoid appearance"

1 Endocrine and Reproductive Physiology

Primary Aldosteronism (Conn's syndrome)
- Caused by excess aldosterone production in the glomerulosa.
- Low K^+, metabolic alkalosis and increase ECF → hypertension.
- Low plasma renin levels.

1.6 Thyroid Hormones

Questions

1. What influences the release of TSH from the anterior pituitary?
   - TRH from the hypothalamus
   - T4 and T3
   - Temperature
   - Stress
   - Dopamine
   - Glucocorticosteroids

2. Which thyroid hormone is released in the greatest quantity?
   93% of the thyroid hormone released from the thyroid is T4, with the remaining amount being T3 with a small amount of rT3.
   However it is T3 that is more potent (4×) and in the periphery 50% of T4 is converted to T3.

3. What is needed for iodide concentration in the thyroid gland?
   Na^+/I^- symporter in the basolateral membrane of thyroid cells. It works by secondary active transport. Energy is provided by the electrochemical gradient of Na^+ which is maintained by Na^+/K^+ ATPase. It has the ability to concentrate iodide to 40× that found in plasma.

4. What percentage of T4 and T3 are bound to plasma proteins?
   T4 and T3 are highly protein bound, 99.98% and 99.8% respectively.

5. What are the clinical features of hypothyroidism and what are some causes?
   Clinical features include:
   - General slowness
   - Husky voice
   - ↑ Cholesterol
   - Sparse dry hair
   - ↓ Reflexes
   - Weight gain

   Causes can be divided into primary [e.g. failure of the thyroid gland (TSH will be high)] or secondary [due to pituitary or hypothalamic disease (TSH will be low)].

Short notes
Thyroid Gland:
Weighs 15–20 g with extensive blood supply.

- Secretes thyroid hormones from thyroid follicles (and calcitonin from parafollicular C cells)
- Thyroid made up of follicles, lined with cuboidal epithelial cells and filled with colloid (mostly thyroglobulin)
- Secretion is under control of TSH, thyrotropin (from anterior pituitary) via TRH (from hypothalamus), with T4 + T3 acting on the pituitary and hypothalamus
    - Higher centres have only a small influence
    - Secretion ↑ with cold; ↓ with ↑ T4, somatostatin, stress, dopamine and glucocorticoids (Fig. 1.4)

Formation and secretion of thyroid hormone:

- Principal hormones released from the thyroid are 93% thyroxine (T4) and 7% triiodothyronine (T3) plus a small amount of rT3
    - T3 is also formed in the peripheral tissues by conversion of T4 → T3
    - T3 is 4× more active than T4
- Iodine Metabolism
    - Ingested iodine is converted to iodide and absorbed
    - Daily requirement is about 150 µg/day, with about 120 µg entering the thyroid

    80 µg is made into hormone, with about 40 µg diffusing into the ECF

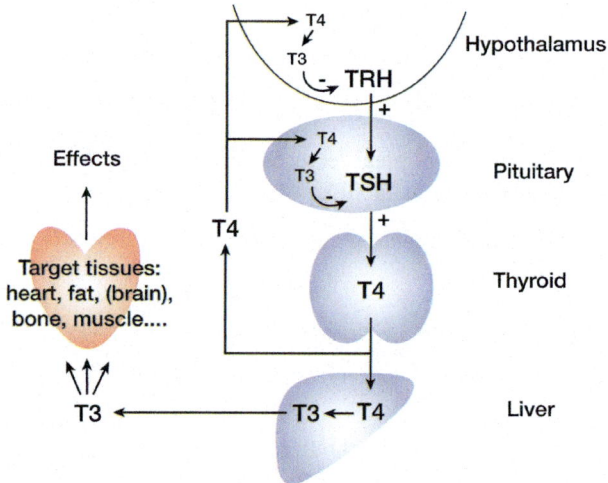

Fig. 1.4 Thyroid hormone release and function

Fig. 1.5 Na⁺/I⁻ symporter

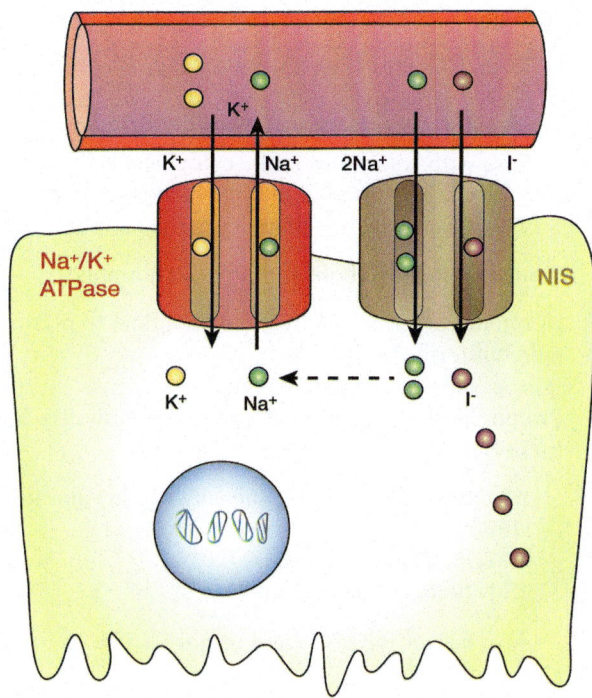

- Na⁺/I⁻ Symporter (Fig. 1.5)
    - Operates via Na⁺/K⁺ ATP-ase which then allows secondary active transport of iodide into the cell

    Concentration gradient of 20–40×
    Rate of iodide uptake is influenced by TSH
- Thyroid hormone synthesis
    - Each thyroglobulin molecule contains ~70 tyrosine amino acids
    - Thyroperoxidase oxidises iodide (blocked by thiourea, propylthiouracil) back into iodine
    - Iodine then enters the colloid and binds to tyrosine residues which are attached to thyroglobulin
    - After synthesis, each thyroglobulin molecule contains 30 thyroxine molecules with less triiodothyronine. (Adequate supply for 3 months)
    - When needed this colloid is ingested into the cells and free T4 and T3 is cleaved off and released into the bloodstream

- Secretion
    - T4 and T3 are cleaved from the thyroglobulin molecule
    - Apical surface of the thyroid cell creates a pseudopod that causes pinocytosis of colloid
    - Fuse with lysosomes in the cytoplasm and proteases release T4 and T3
    - T4 and T3 diffuse out into the bloodstream
    - 93% T4 and 7% T3, however in the periphery 50% of T4 is converted to T3

Transport and metabolism of thyroid hormones:

- Hormones are secreted free and then bind to plasma proteins, which provides a more uniform distribution
- It is only the free component that is active
- Protein binding includes albumin, transthyretin and thyroxine-binding globulin (TBG)
    - Albumin has the largest capacity to carry hormones, but TBG has the highest affinity
    - T4 is extensively bound 99.98%
    - T3 is bound at about 99.8%

    Also has a shorter t ½ and is more active on the tissues

    - TBG levels ↑ with oestrogen and pregnancy, and ↓ with androgens
- Metabolism results from deiodination in the liver, kidneys and other organs
- Much more rT3 and less T3 is formed in fetal life → switches after birth

Effects of thyroid hormones:

- Thyroid hormone receptor (T3 > T4) are either attached to DNA strands or in close proximity
- Calorigenic mechanism → ↑ O_2 consumption in almost all metabolically active tissues (except brain, testes, uterus, anterior pituitary)
- Effect due to ↑ fatty acid metabolism and ↑ in Na^+/K^+ ATP-ase activity
    - CVS- ↑ CO, HR, contractility, blood sugar
    - CNS- ↑ electrical activity and irritability
    - MSK- muscle wasting, tremor
    - GIT- ↑ absorption and fluctuations in carbohydrate metabolism, ↑ Na^+ excretion, ↑ fat metabolism
    - Liver- ↓ cholesterol, phospholipids and triglycerides, ↑ fatty acids, ↑ gluconeogenesis
    - Resp- ↑ RR
    - Other endocrine glands- ↑ insulin, ↑ PTH, ↑ glucocorticoids
    - Growth ↑ → early differentiation, ↓ → slow growth, ↑ erythropoiesis, and accentuates catecholamines

1 Endocrine and Reproductive Physiology

Clinical correlation:

- Hypothyroidism
  - Primary → due to failure of the thyroid gland (TSH will be high)
  - Secondary → due to pituitary or hypothalamic disease (TSH will be low)
  - Features: general slowness, carotenemia, husky voice, ↑ cholesterol, sparse dry hair, ↓ reflexes, weight gain
  - Cretinism: Hypothyroid from birth → ↓ growth, ↓ mentation; may be from thyroid agenesis, genetic cause of ↓ I^-

- Hyperthyroidism
  - Graves' disease (auto-immune), toxic multinodular goiter (TMNG), 2° to higher dysfunction, thyroiditis, ectopic tissue, exogenous hormone
  - Features: Nervousness, tremor, ↑ basal metabolic rate (BMR), warm skin, ↑ HR, ↑ pulse pressure, AF, weight loss, diarrhoea. Note exophthalmos only with Graves' disease.

1.7 Calcium and Phosphate Metabolism

Questions

1. What percentage of calcium is in the ECF?
   0.1%.

2. What are the effects of hypo and hyper-calcaemia?
   Hypocalcaemia causes increased neuronal excitability (e.g. tetany).
   Hypercalcaemia causes CNS depression, shortens QTc, renal stones, constipation.

3. What are the effects of PTH on Ca^{2+} and PO_4 levels in the blood?
   PTH: ↑ plasma Ca^{2+}, ↓plasma PO_4.

   Ca^{2+}

   - Bone- ↑ bone reabsorption → ↑ Ca^{2+}
   - Kidney- ↑ reabsorption of Ca^{2+} in the renal tubule → ↑ Ca^{2+} (although if Ca^{2+} concentration is too high this system may be overwhelmed and renal secretion may increase)
   - GI tract- PTH also increases formation of 1,25 DHCC → ↑ GI Ca^{2+} reabsorption

   PO_4

   - Bone- ↑ bone reabsorption → ↑ PO_4
   - Kidney- ↑ PO_4 excretion in the urine, due to ↓ reabsorption of PO_4 in the proximal tubules
   - GI tract- ↑ absorption from the GIT by increasing formation of 1,25 DHCC in the kidneys.

4. Explain the different changes to Ca^{2+}, PTH and PO_4 with primary, secondary and tertiary hyperparathyroidism.

	Primary hyperparathyroidism	Secondary hyperparathyroidism	Tertiary hyperparathyroidism
Calcium	↑	↓/N	↑
Parathyroid hormone	↑	↑	↑↑
Phosphate	↓	↑/N	↑

5. What cells of the thyroid release calcitonin?
   The parafollicular C cells which make up only 0.1% of the human thyroid gland and are remnants of the ultimobranchial body.

6. What level does Ca^{2+} need to be to stimulate release of calcitonin?
   It needs to be above 2.4 mmol/L. It acts to lower Ca^{2+} level by inhibiting bone reabsorption, ↓ absorbtion and ↑ urinary excretion.

Short notes
Calcium

- Total body stores = 1.3 kg (99% skeleton, 1% intracellular, 0.1% ECF). 'Exchangeable calcium' is about 0.4–1% of total body calcium (TBC).
- Calcium balance → Dietary intake ~25 mmol; net absorption 3 mmol;
    - Bone change over 500 mmol; cell mediated bone turnover 7 mmol
    - Glomerular filtrate 250 mmol; reabsorbed 247 mmol; excreted 3 mmol
- Absorption
    - Active absorption in duodenum and upper jejunum (calcitriol dependent)
    - Small amount further down GI tract, which is passive
    - Impaired by phosphates, oxalates, fatty acids → form insoluble Ca^{2+} compounds
    - 90% of calcium intake is excreted in faeces.
- Plasma calcium
    - 45% is protein bound (albumin);

    pH dependent: <u>Acidosis</u> → ↓ binding → more free Ca^{2+}. <u>Alkalosis</u> → ↑ binding → less free Ca^{2+}→ tetany

    - 45% is ionised (active fraction and regulated)
    - 10% in various complexes
    - Hypocalcaemia causes increased neuronal excitability (e.g. tetany).
    - Hypercalcaemia causes CNS depression, shortens QTc, renal stones, constipation

- Urinary excretion
    - Ionised and complexed Ca^{2+} is filtered, 99% absorbed

    60% in the proximal tubule
    40% in the ascending limb of loop of Henle and distal tubule

    PTH stimulates reabsorption in the distal tubule, increased reabsorption with ↓ plasma $[Ca^{2+}]$.

Phosphate

- Total body stores = 700 g (85% skeleton, significant amount in cellular molecules), plasma concentration ~1.2 mmol/L but this varies
- Absorption is dependent on dietary intake, almost all dietary PO_4 is absorbed into the blood, calcitriol stimulates absorption
- Urinary excretion
    - 85–90% of filtered PO_4 is reabsorbed in the proximal tubule. This is inhibited by PTH.

Bone

- Bone organic matrix is strengthened by calcium salts
    - Organic matrix is collagen (95%) with ground substance (5%) (extracellular fluid + proteoglycans e.g. hyaluronic acid)
    - Ground salt is composed of hydroxyapatite $[Ca_{10}(PO_4)_6(OH)_2]$.
- Bone production: Osteoblasts secrete collagen and ground substance to make osteoid. Some of the osteoblasts get caught in osteoid → osteocytes. Calcium precipitates onto osteoid → hydroxyapatite.
- Bone resorption by osteoclasts which secrete proteolytic enzymes and acid.
- Acts as a buffer for plasma Ca^{2+} levels.

Parathyroid glands (usually 4, superior and inferior on each side)

- Each gland is a richly vascularised disk (3 × 6 × 2 mm) containing two types of cells;
    - Chief cells – majority, contain a prominent golgi apparatus, ER and secretory granules → PTH
    - Oxyphil cells – minority, but larger, unknown function

Synthesis and metabolism of PTH

- Synthesised by chief cells
- Linear polypeptide (MW 9500; 84 amino acids); PreproPTH → ER → ProPTH → PTH secretory granules
- Normal plasma level is 10–55 pg/mL, t ½ of 10 min, cleared by the kidneys
- Secretion ↑ by
    - Low Ca^{2+}, low Mg^{2+}, high PO_4

- Secretion ↓ by
  - High Ca^{2+}, high Mg^{2+}, calcitriol

Actions of PTH (Fig. 1.6)

- Increases plasma Ca^{2+}, decreases plasma PO_4
- Ca^{2+} - acts directly on bone to increase bone reabsorption and mobilise Ca^{2+}
  - Also increases the reabsorption of Ca^{2+} in the renal tubules, although if Ca^{2+} concentration is too high this system may be overwhelmed and renal secretion may increase
  - PTH also increases formation of 1,25 DHCC → increases GI Ca^{2+} reabsorption
- PO_4 - increases Ca^{2+} release from bone, increases PO_4 excretion in the urine, due to decreased reabsorption of PO_4 in the proximal tubules
- Increased absorption from the GI tract by increasing formation of 1,25 DHCC in the kidneys.
- Mild acidosis
- Even though Ca^{2+} reabsorption is ↑, more is filtered, therefore often more shows up in the urine
- Long-term, PTH stimulates osteoblasts and osteoclasts

Mechanism of action

- Probably three different receptors
  - G2 coupled → adenyl cyclase → increases intracellular cAMP

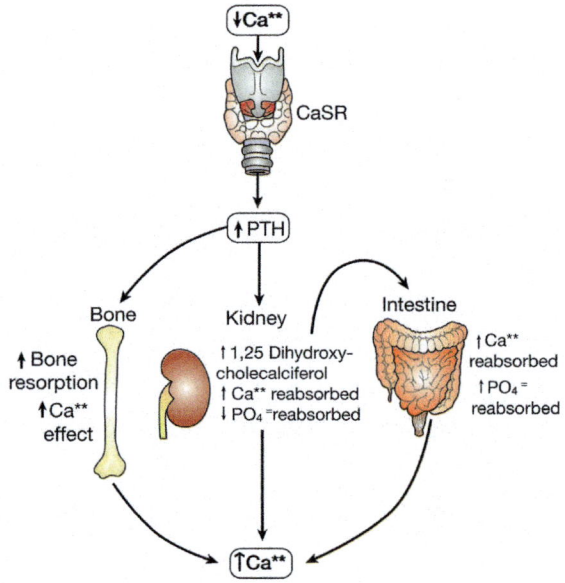

Fig. 1.6 PTH release and function

Regulation of secretion

- Circulating ionised Ca^{2+} acts directly on the PTH glands in a negative feedback fashion
    - Key is cell membrane GPCR Ca^{2+} receptor 'calcium sensing receptor' → inhibits PTH secretion
    - If Ca^{2+} is high → PTH secretion is inhibited → Ca^{2+} is deposited in bones
    - If Ca^{2+} is low → PTH is secreted → Ca^{2+} is mobilised
    - 1,25 DHCC → decreases preproPTH mRNA
    - Increased plasma PO_4 → stimulates secretion
    - Mg^{2+} is required in the process

Calcitriol (Vit D)

- Formation: Cholesterols → UV light → Vit D3 → liver → 25 HC (t ½ of 12 days) → 1,25 DHCC
    - Last step stimulated by PTH, ↓ Ca^{2+}, prolactin, GH, calcitonin and ↓ by opposites incl. acidosis
- Actions: Largely through the GI tract. Binds to nuclear receptors → modifies DNA/RNA
    - ↑ gut uptake, ↑ reabsorption, ↑ osteocyte change, ↓ Ca^{2+} and PO_4 excretion, provides negative feedback to PTH

Calcitonin

- Produced by the parafollicular cells of the thyroid
- Stimulated by ↑ Ca^{2+} (>2.4 mmol/L) as well as gastrin.
- Action is ↓ Ca^{2+} AND ↓ PO_4, by inhibiting bone reabsorption, decreasing absorption and ↑ urinary excretion

Others

- Glucocorticoids inhibit bone formation and gut absorption (through vitamin D)
- GH stimulates vitamin D formation → ↑ Ca^{2+} and ↑ PO_4
- ↑ thyroid hormones can increase Ca^{2+} levels (also causes hypercalcuria and osteoporosis)

Features of hypercalcemia

- Weakness and constipation → due to ↓ muscular excitability
- Polyuria → due to inhibition of ADH, and dehydration
- Renal calculi, hypertension, cardiac arrhythmias, psychological disturbances
- Peptic ulceration → from ↑ gastric acid 2° to ↑ Ca^{2+}

Causes of hypercalcemia

- Hyperparathyroidism
- Malignancy (PTHrP, multiple myeloma, bone metastasis)
- Sarcoidosis ($\uparrow$ Vitamin D)
- Thiazide diuretics (stimulate Ca^{2+} reabsorption)
- Thyrotoxicosis
- Paget's disease

Features and causes of hypocalcaemia

- Tetany ($\uparrow$ excitability), numbness, stridor, cataracts, psychological disturbances
- Transiently post-op, pancreatitis, prolonged hypoparathyroidism, malabsorption and CRF

CRF

- $\downarrow$ renal function $\rightarrow$ $\uparrow$ plasma PO_4, $\downarrow$ vitamin D production $\rightarrow$ $\downarrow\downarrow Ca^{2+}$
    - $\rightarrow$ 2° hyperparathyroidism $\rightarrow$ $\uparrow$ bone reabsorption with $\uparrow$ ALP and ectopic calcification

Effects of parathyroidectomy

- PTH is essential for life. Following parathyroidectomy there is a steady decline in plasma Ca^{2+}
    - If so $\rightarrow$ neuromuscular hyperexcitability $\rightarrow$ hypocalcaemic tetany
- Symptoms usually develop 2–3 days post-operatively, but may be delayed
- Chvostek's and Trousseau's signs
- Treat with Calcium +/− Vitamin D replacement

Parathyroid excess (PTH injections/ adenomas)

- Characterised by hypercalcemia and hypophosphatemia
- In chronic renal disease $\rightarrow$ low Ca^{2+} $\rightarrow$ 2° hyperparathyroidism develops
- PTHrP is produced by a number of tissues and is necessary for survival
    - In malignancy hypercalcemia is common due to ectopic PTHrP secretion. This may be due to bone metastasis (20%) or due to elevated levels of PTHrP (80% - breast, kidney, ovary, skin)

	Primary hyperparathyroidism	Secondary hyperparathyroidism	Tertiary hyperparathyroidism
Calcium	$\uparrow$	$\downarrow$/N	$\uparrow$
Parathyroid hormone	$\uparrow$	$\uparrow$	$\uparrow\uparrow$
Phosphate	$\downarrow$	$\uparrow$/N	$\uparrow$

1 Endocrine and Reproductive Physiology

1.8 Glucoregulatory Hormones

Questions

1. Name the types of cells found in the islets of Langerhans.
   Three types of cells in the islets of Langerhans
   Alpha – glucagon (25%);
   Beta – insulin and amylin (60%);
   Delta – somatostatin (10%).

2. What is the main effect of insulin?
   It is secreted primarily in response to hyperglycaemia and acts to increase muscle cell uptake of glucose, as without insulin they are relatively impermeable to glucose and use fatty acids as their primary fuel.

3. How is insulin released from the pancreas?
   Raised glucose levels → Glut-2 → Enters β cells→ ↑ ATP → closes K^+ channels → depolarisation → opens Ca^{2+} channels → Ca^{2+} enters the cells → triggers exocytosis of insulin

4. What effect does insulin have on fat metabolism?
   Activation of lipoprotein lipase in the capillary walls of the adipose tissue, inhibition of hormone-sensitive lipase.

5. What is the consequence of insulin deficiency?
   - Glucose- reduced entry of glucose into peripheral cells and ↑ plasma glucose
   - Protein- ↑ rate at which amino acids are catabolised → protein deficiency
   - Fatty acids- Fat breakdown → ketosis → acidosis → coma
   - Poor resistance to infections

6. Name 4 stimuli for the release of glucagon?

Any of the following:

- Hypoglycaemia
- Amino acids
- Cholecystokinin (CCK)
- Gastrin
- Cortisol
- Exercise
- Stress
- Infection
- Theophylline

7. What is the action of glucagon?

- Primarily on the liver by stimulating glycogen breakdown via glycogenolysis and glucose production via gluconeogenesis
- In fat and liver, stimulates lipolysis via action of hormone-sensitive lipase (adipose and liver), ketosis, inotropic effect on the heart, ↑ insulin secretion
- Has **NO** effect on muscle

8. What is the most important hormone in the defense of acute hypoglycaemia?

Adrenaline.

Short notes

Pancreas: Three types of cells in the islets of Langerhans
1. Alpha – glucagon (25%)
2. Beta – insulin and amylin (60%)
3. Delta – somatostatin (10%) (Fig. 1.7).

Glucose

- Levels are normally very closely controlled
- Entry via intestinal absorption, glycogen breakdown (liver) and gluconeogenesis (liver and kidney)
- Utilised in all tissues (muscle, brain, adipose, RBC and kidney)
- Controlling hormones are insulin, glucagon, somatostatin, pancreatic polypeptide

Insulin (storing hormone when there is excess energy)

- Preproinsulin → proinsulin (stored in granules) → insulin in β-pancreatic islet cells
- Secretion occurs by exocytosis in response to ↑ intracellular Ca^{2+}
- Stimulation
    - Blood glucose above 5 mmol/L → secretion ↑ rapidly
    - Glucose → GLUT-2 → Enters β cells → ↑ ATP → closes K^+ channels → depolarisation → opens Ca^{2+} channels → Ca^{2+} enters the cells → triggers exocytosis of insulin

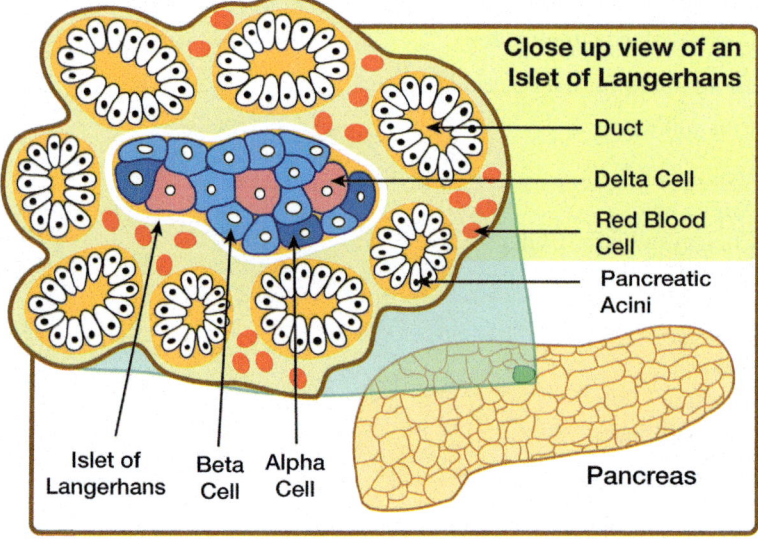

Fig. 1.7 Islets of Langerhans

- Other triggers
  - Arginine, leucine and other amino acids
  - Cyclic AMP, note that Adrenaline lowers cAMP → inhibits insulin release
  - Glucagon and theophylline via cAMP
  - Autonomic stimulation via acetylcholine
  - GI hormones (**GIP**, + enteroglucagon, secretin, CCK)
  - Oral hypoglycaemic drugs → close ATP sensitive K^+ channels
- Inhibitors of insulin secretion
  - Somatostatin, beta blockers, K^+ depletion, thiazide diuretics [negative feedback]
- Secreted into the portal vein, hence liver is exposed to higher levels
- Effects → hormone of fuel storage and anabolism. Primary action is to increase glucose uptake in muscles.
  - Adipose tissue: ↑ glucose entry, ↑ fatty acid synthesis, ↑ triglyceride deposition, activation of lipoprotein lipase, ↑ K^+ uptake
  - Muscle: ↑ glucose entry, ↑ glycogen entry, ↑ amino acids uptake, ↑ protein synthesis, ↑ protein catabolism,
  - Liver: ↓ ketogenesis, ↑ protein synthesis, ↑ lipid synthesis, ↓ glucose output
  - General: ↑ cell growth
  - Stimulates whole body glucose uptake (skeletal muscle, heart muscle, smooth muscle and adipose tissue)

    Some tissues do not respond (brain, gut, RBC, pancreatic β-cells)
- Consequences of deficiency
  - Diabetes mellitus (reduced entry of glucose into peripheral cells and ↑ plasma glucose)
  - ↑ rate at which amino acids are catabolised
  - Protein deficiency and poor resistance to infections
  - Ketosis → acidosis → coma

Glucagon (glucose mobilising hormone)

- Preproglucagon → Glucagon; occurs in α-pancreatic islet cells
- Stimulation
  - Hypoglycaemia, amino acids, CCK, gastrin, cortisol, exercise, stress, infection, beta adrenergic, theophylline
- Inhibition
  - Glucose (seems to require insulin), somatostatin, secretin, free fatty acids, ketones, insulin, GABA, alpha stimulators

- Actions
    - Primarily on the liver by stimulating glycogen breakdown and gluconeogenesis.
    - In other tissues it stimulates lipolysis via action of hormone sensitive lipase (adipose and liver), ketosis, inotropic effect on the heart, ↑ insulin secretion
    - Has **NO** effect on muscle

Somatostatin

- From D-cells → Two forms
- Inhibit insulin, glucagon, pancreatic polypeptide and can also inhibit GB contraction (by ↓ CCK release)

Pancreatic polypeptide

- Released from F-cells after a protein meal

Other hormones having effect:

- Catecholamines: The most important defence against acute hypoglycaemia
↑ liver glycogenolysis, ↓ Glucose uptake, ↑ circulating FFA with no effect on protein synthesis
Thyroid hormones: increase absorption of glucose from the intestine, ↑ liver glycogenolysis
- Glucocorticoids ↑ blood glucose, ↑ protein breakdown, insulin resistance
- Growth hormone: 'Diabetogenic' mobilising free fatty acids, inhibiting glucose utilisation and inhibiting insulin receptor function

Overall insulin lowers blood glucose, others raise it.
Insulin

- In fasting protects against ↑ catabolism (↓ gluconeogenesis, ↓ lipolysis, ↓ protein breakdown, ↓ hepatic ketogenesis
- After feeding is strongly anabolic → promotes storage

Glucagon

- In fasting, exercise or stress it helps to maintain blood glucose by;
    - ↑ glycogen breakdown, and ↑ glucose formation, and sets up liver for ketone production.
    - After a protein meal it protects against insulin induced hypoglycaemia

Adrenaline

- Is the most important defence against acute hypoglycaemia
    - ↓ Glucose uptake
    - ↑ Hepatic formation
    - ↓ Insulin release
    - ↑ Lipolysis and provides FFA

1 Endocrine and Reproductive Physiology

Cortisol
- Promotes peripheral tissue breakdown and antagonises insulin

GH
- ↑ anabolism and ↓ catabolism, inhibits insulin effect, stimulates lipolysis

Thyroid hormone
- Stimulates lipolysis and ↑ blood glucose

1.9 Female Hormones

Questions

1. Which cells of the ovary secrete oestrogen?
   Granulosa and theca interna cells.

2. Explain the effects of LH and FSH.
   FSH causes growth of follicles and LH surge stimulates ovulation.
   FSH: Stimulates growth of 6–12 primary follicles. It also allows for growth of granulosa, theca interna and externa cells. Granulosa cells have FSH and then LH receptors.
   LH: Main hormone for ovulation and necessary for the final development of the follicle. Theca interna cells have LH receptors and NOT FSH receptors.

   (a) Stimulates the release of oestrogen from the theca interna.
   (b) LH appears to stimulate the granulosa and theca interna cells into a progesterone secreting type of cell.

3. On which day of the menstrual cycle does ovulation occur?
   Day 14 after the onset of menstruation.

4. What effects does oestrogen have?

   (a) At puberty increases size of female sex organs
   (b) Uterus and vagina

   - Changes cuboidal epithelium to squamous in the vagina
   - Increases the amount of uterine muscle and increases the content of contractile proteins
   - Sensitises the myometrium to oxytocin

   (c) Breast

   - Development of stromal tissue, extensive ductal system and deposition of fat
   - Breast enlargement during pregnancy

(d) Other
- Inhibits osteoclastic activity (osteoporosis after menopause)
- Increases secretion of angiotensinogen
- Slightly increases protein deposition
- Increases metabolism and fat deposition
- Soft skin with increased vascularity

5. Can theca cells convert androgens to oestrogens?
   No, as they lack the enzyme aromatase.
6. Why does osteoporosis occur after menopause?
   Oestrogen inhibits osteoclastic activity. After menopause, no oestrogen is secreted by the ovaries, hence there is an increase in bone turnover.
7. Where does fertilisation of the ovum occur?
   Typically in the ampulla of the fallopian tube.
8. What mechanisms increase oxygen carriage in the fetus in the setting of low placental PaO_2?
   1. HbF causes left shift of the oxygen dissociation curve
   2. Higher Hb concentration in fetus
9. What effect does oestrogen and progesterone have on the breast?
   Oestrogens are primarily responsible for duct development and progesterone for lobular development in the breast.

Short notes
Menstrual cycle: (Fig. 1.8)
Control from Hypothalamus (GnRH), released in pulse q90m → Anterior pituitary (FSH and LH) → Ovary (Progesterone and Oestrogen)
FSH: Stimulates accelerated growth of 6–12 primary follicles with rapid proliferation of granulosa cells as well as a second class of cells that form the theca interna and externa. Granulosa cells have FSH and then LH receptors.
LH: Main hormone for ovulation and necessary for the final development of the follicle. Theca interna cells have LH receptors and **NOT** FSH receptors.

- LH appears to stimulate the granulosa and theca interna cells into a progesterone secreting type of cell
  Ovarian hormones:
  Transported bound to proteins - Albumin + oestrogen and progesterone-binding globulins
  Oestrogen - β-oestradiol (most potent), oestrone and oestriol. During menstrual cycle peak conc ~24–48 h preceding ovulation.
  Release: In non pregnant women released only by the ovaries

- In pregnant women also placenta

  Effects:

- At puberty increases size of female sex organs

1 Endocrine and Reproductive Physiology

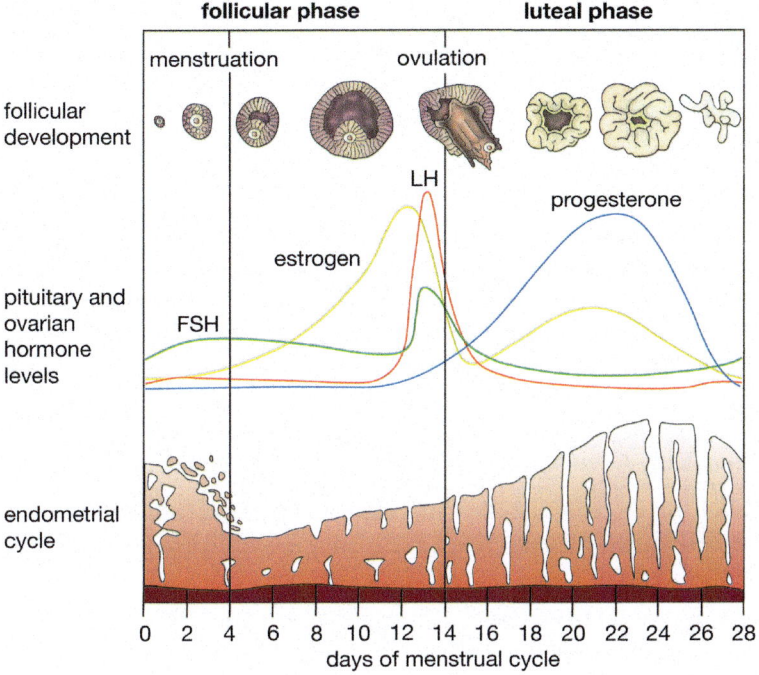

Fig. 1.8 Menstrual cycle

- Uterus and vagina
  - Changes cuboidal epithelium to squamous in the vagina
  - Increases the amount of uterine muscle and increases the content of contractile proteins
  - Sensitises the myometrium to oxytocin
- Breast
  - Development of stromal tissue, extensive ductal system and deposition of fat
  - Breast enlargement during pregnancy
- Other
  - Inhibits osteoclastic activity (osteoporosis after menopause)
  - Increases secretion of angiotensinogen
  - Slightly increases protein deposition
  - Increases metabolism and fat deposition
  - Soft skin with increased vascularity

Excretion: Conjugated in the liver; 1/5 bile; 4/5 kidneys. Liver converts oestrogen to non-potent oestriol

Progesterone – Peak concentration at day 21 of the menstrual cycle
Release: In non pregnant women only in latter half of ovarian cycle. In pregnancy- Secreted by both corpus luteum and placenta.
Effects:

- Uterus and vagina
  - Decreases the response of uterus to oxytocin
  - Progesterone induces the secretion of thick, tenacious cervical mucous
  - Fallopian tubes secretory changes of mucosa
  - Promotes secretory changes in the uterine endometrium in the latter half of pregnancy

- Breast
  - Stimulates development of breast lobules and alveoli

Metabolism: Degraded to other steroids with no progesterone effect in minutes
Menstrual cycle – 28 days
Follicular phase:

- FSH (mostly) and LH induce growth of 6–12 primary follicles with rapid proliferation of the granulosa cells and outer theca layer [theca interna (hormone release) and externa (vascular capsule)]
- Granulosa cells secrete follicular fluid into the antrum, which is high in oestrogen.
- Only one follicle fully matures and the remainder undergo atresia.
- LH is necessary for final follicular growth and concentration increase 6–10× 2 days prior to ovulation. It also converts granulosa and theca interna cells to progesterone secreting cells.

Luteal phase:

- After ovulation there is 'luteinisation' of granulosa and theca interna cells as they become filled with lipid inclusions.
- Granulosa cells produce progesterone and oestrogen.
- Theca cells form androgens—androstenedione and testosterone (However in granulosa cells most are converted to oestrogen by aromatase).

Corpus luteum - prepares a receptive endometrium for the fertilised ovum. If ovum not fertilised then the corpus luteum involutes, removing feedback inhibition of anterior pituitary and menstruation occurs.
Also known as the; **Proliferative** phase (oestrogen), stromal and epithelial cells proliferate rapidly. **Secretory** phase (progesterone), swelling and secretory development.

Pregnancy -
Ovum (primary oocyte) → released from ovarian follicle surrounded by corona radiata (secondary oocyte 23C + first polar body) → fallopian tube (fertilisation most commonly in ampulla) → sperm penetrate the corona radiata and the zona pellucida → mature ovum + second polar body + sperm = fertilised ovum or zygote. After implantation, ongoing nutrition of this conceptus is dependent on corpus luteum secretion of progesterone, oestrogen and relaxin. After about 6 weeks the placenta is able to produce enough oestrogen and progesterone to maintain pregnancy. If a mother has an oophorectomy < 6 weeks it will lead to miscarriage.
Oxygen diffusion in the placenta: Low PaO_2 however HbF has a left shift, higher Hb concentration in fetus.
Hormones in pregnancy: Initially secreted by the corpus luteum under stimulation of hCG from the developing placenta, later on the placenta takes over (Fig. 1.9).

- Human chorionic gonadotropin - prevents involution of the corpus luteum with fertilisation to encourage oestrogen and progesterone secretion. Measured in blood 8–9 days after ovulation.
- Oestrogen function: Enlargement of uterus, enlargement of breasts and growth of ductal structures, enlargement of external genitalia, relaxation of pelvic ligaments.
- Progesterone function: Development of decidual cells in the uterine endometrium, decrease contractility of uterus, lobule breast development.
- Human chorionic somatomammotrophin: <u>Function is uncertain</u>

Breast:

- Prolactin is the most important hormone for the release of milk into the alveoli
- Oestrogens are primarily responsible for duct development and progesterone for lobular development in the breast. The drop in oestrogen after birth is responsible for initiation of lactation.
- Oxytocin is responsible for milk let down

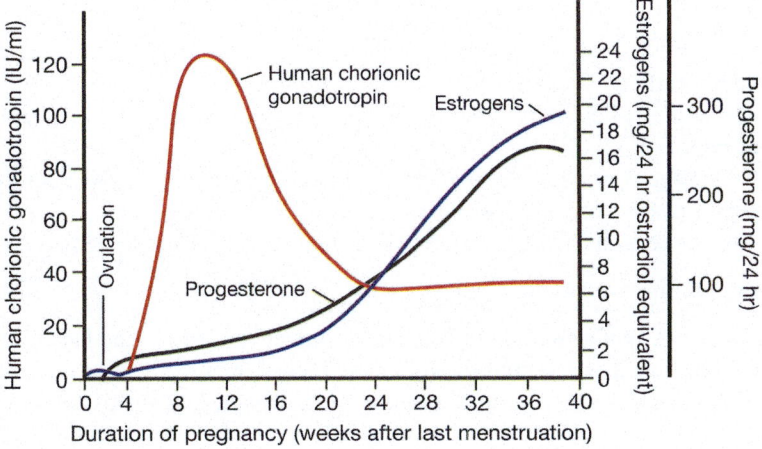

Fig. 1.9 Hormones in pregnancy

1.10 Male Hormones

Questions

1. Which hormones are involved in spermatogenesis?
   Testosterone, LH, FSH, oestrogen and GH (*see short notes*).

2. What is the most potent androgen?
   DHEA

3. At which age do males secrete testosterone?
   The Leydig cells, which secrete testosterone, are under control of LH from the anterior pituitary and are active for the first few months of life and after puberty. Virtually no testosterone is produced between the ages of 2–3 months to puberty.

4. What hormones do Leydig and Sertoli cells release?
   Leydig – testosterone
   Sertoli – inhibin

   Short notes
   Sex differentiation

- Y-chromosome determines the male sex, with a gene on the short arm of the Y-chromosome producing Testis Determining Factor (TDF). TDF → male. No TDF → female.
- Until 6 weeks the gonad remains undifferentiated
    - Male: Wolffian duct plus mesonephros becomes the epididymis, the vas deferens, and the seminal vesicle.
    - Female: Mullerian ligament forms the uterine tubes, uterus, cervix, and the upper two third of the vagina.
- Testosterone and Mullerian Inhibitory Factor cause regression of the female parts
    - Turners (45XO) → develop female external and internal genitalia, but ovaries do not fully develop
    - Klinefelter (47XXY) → develop male genitalia but the testes do not fully develop
    - ↑ Androgens in a female → female genitalia internally (no MIF) but external genitalia are masculinised
    - ↓ Androgens in a male → male gonads but external genitalia remain female

   Hormones involved in spermatogenesis;

1. Testosterone, synthesised by Leydig cells from cholesterol, located in the interstitium of the testis, is essential for growth and division of the testicular germ cells.
2. Luteinising hormone (anterior pituitary) → Leydig cells → testosterone

3. Follicle stimulating hormone (anterior pituitary) → Sertoli cells → spermatogenesis
4. Oestrogen → formed from testosterone in the Sertoli cells
5. Growth hormone → controls metabolic functions of the testes (Fig. 1.10).

Androgens:
Secreted by the leydig cells (20% mass of testicle) under control of LH from the anterior pituitary. 98% protein bound (65% to GBG, 33% to albumin).
Testes secrete testosterone, dihydrotestosterone and androstenedione.
Testosterone is the most abundant, but converted to more potent dihydrotestosterone in target tissues by 5 alpha reductase.
Effects of testosterone after puberty

- Increases musculature and bone deposition
- Increases basal metabolic rate (BMR)
- RBC and ECF
- Body hair distribution
- Voice changes
- Increases skin thickness
- Acne

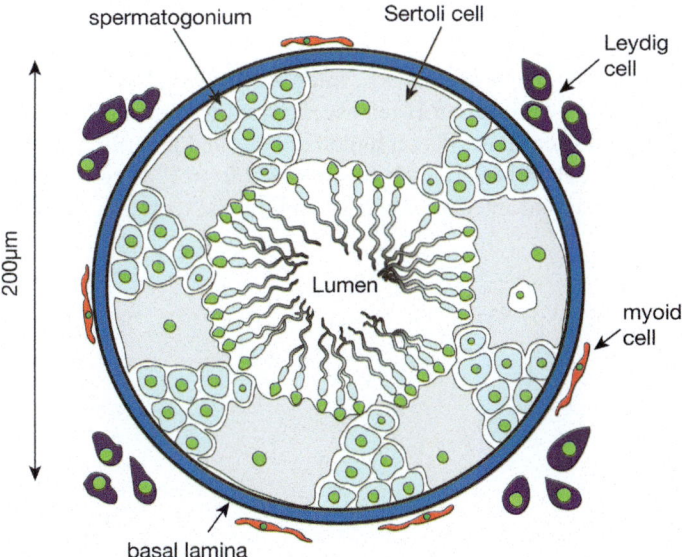

Fig. 1.10 Spermatogenesis

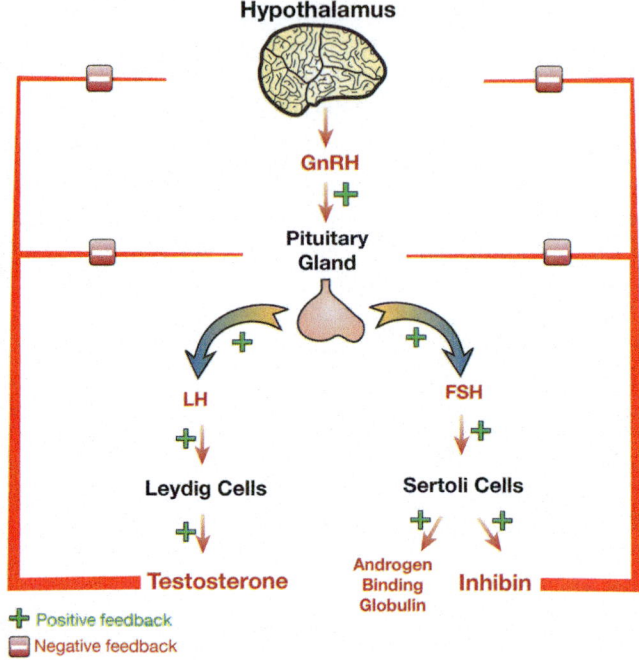

Fig. 1.11 Gonadotropin cycle

Release: GnRH (hypothalamus) intermittent release → release from Gonadotrophin cells – pulsatile LH release, FSH only slight fluctuations.

Inhibition: Testosterone works on hypothalamus and anterior pituitary to inhibit release of GnRH, LH and FSH. Inhibin is released from FSH cells and acts directly on the hypothalamus and anterior pituitary to inhibit the secretion of FSH (Fig. 1.11).

Chapter 2
Gastrointestinal Physiology

S. Ali Mirjalili, Lucy Hinton, and Simon Richards

2.1 Gastrointestinal Function

Questions

1. What type of movements occur in the GI tract?
   Propulsion and mixing.
   Propulsive movements occur via peristalsis. The usual stimulus is distension but also irritants and parasympathetic supply. Requires an active myenteric plexus. It is directed towards the anus. Downstream gut typically relaxes to accommodate the bolus.
   Mixing movements. Constricting type actions, produces mixing if against a closed sphincter.

2. What volume of secretions are produced in each area of the gastrointestinal tract (day/mL) and how much is reabsorbed? (Fig. 2.1)

3. What are the three mechanisms of absorption in the gut?
   (1) Active transport, (2) Diffusion, (3) Solvent drag

4. Name the layers of the bowel wall (outer to inner)
   (1) Serosa (2) Longitudinal muscle layer (3) Circular muscle layer (4) Submucosa (5) Mucosa

---

S. A. Mirjalili (✉)
Department of Anatomy and Medical Imaging, University of Auckland, Auckland, New Zealand
e-mail: a.mirjalili@auckland.ac.nz

L. Hinton
Department of General Surgery, Tauranga Hospital, Tauranga, New Zealand

S. Richards
Department of General Surgery, University of Otago, Christchurch, New Zealand

Christchurch Hospital, Christchurch, New Zealand

© Springer Nature Singapore Pte Ltd. and People's Medical Publishing House Co. Ltd. 2019
S. A. Mirjalili (ed.), *Physiology for General Surgical Sciences Examination (GSSE)*, https://doi.org/10.1007/978-981-13-2580-9_2

Daily water turnover (mL) in the gastrointestinal tract		
Ingested		2000
Endogenous secretions		7000
Salivary glands	1500	
Stomach	2500	
Bile	500	
Pancreas	1500	
Intestine	+1000	
	7000	
Total input		9000
Reabsorbed		8800
Jejunum	5500	
Ileum	2000	
Colon	+1300	
	8800	
Balance in stool		200

Fig. 2.1 Fluid balance in digestive tract

Short notes

- Bowel wall made up of (1) Serosa (2) Longitudinal muscle layer (3) Circular muscle layer (4) Submucosa (5) Mucosa
  - Muscularis mucosae lies in the deepest layer of the mucosa just above submucosa
  - Gastrointestinal (GI) smooth muscle acts as a syncytium
- GI smooth muscle is excited intrinsically by slow waves and spikes.
- Basic electrical rhythm (BER) caused by interstitial cells of Cajal.
  - Slow waves are undulating changes in membrane potential (stomach 4/min, duodenum 12/min, ileum 8/min, caecum 2/min, sigmoid 8/min)
  - Spike potential are true action potentials (through Ca^{2+} ions)
    - A number of factors make it more excitable (stretch, acetylcholine, parasympathetic supply and hormones)
  - Some muscle exhibits tonic contraction
- Enteric nervous system (ENS) extends from cranial to caudal, and is composed of:
  - Outer, myenteric plexus (Auerbach's plexus) which largely controls GI movement
  - Inner, submucosal plexus (Meissner's plexus) which largely controls secretion and local GI blood flow
  - Acetylcholine almost always excites GI activity, norepinephrine almost always inhibits

- Parasympathetic supply is via cranial (vagus) and sacral (S2-4) divisions, and generally enhances GI function
  - Postganglionic neurons of the parasympathetic system are located in the above plexuses
- Sympathetic supply passes to ganglia and postganglionic fibres continue on to the gut
  - Inhibits many of the neurons by directly releasing norepinephrine
- Afferent supply is rich and passes to local ganglia before continuing to the brain stem
- GI reflexes may be
  - Integrated entirely within the enteric nervous system (peristalsis)
  - To the prevertebral sympathetic ganglia (gastrocolic, enterogastric, colonoileal reflexes)
  - To the spinal cord or brain stem (defecation reflexes)

Two types of movements - mixing and propulsion.

- Propulsive movements occur via peristalsis.
  - The usual stimulus is distension but also irritants and parasympathetic supply.
  - Requires an active myenteric plexus which is directed towards the anus.
  - Downstream gut typically relaxes to accommodate the bolus.
- Mixing movements. Constricting type actions produce mixing if against a closed sphincter.

GI blood flow – The Splanchnic Circulation

- Blood from the gut, spleen, pancreas passes through the liver → the portal vein → millions of sinusoids → hepatic veins
- Blood flow increases significantly with increased GI work
  - Vasodilator substances are released in the digestive process (Cholecystokinin (CCK), vasoactive intestinal polypeptide (VIP), gastrin, secretin)
  - Release of kinins into the gut wall
  - Local hypoxia from increased activity
- The normal blood supply into a villus forms a counter current system – can lead to villus ischaemia in setting of hypoperfusion
- Parasympathetic stimulation increases blood flow. Sympathetic does the opposite.
- The gut can also act as a significant blood reservoir.

Approximately 2 L of water is ingested each day. About 7 L of fluid is also secreted from salivary glands, gastric glands, pancreas, liver and small intestine into the GI tract. Of the 9 L of fluid entering the GI tract, 7.5 L is reabsorbed, leaving approximately 1.5 L to pass into the colon. A small amount of fluid (200 mL) is normally lost in the faeces and the remaining is reabsorbed into the blood.

- The stomach generally has very poor absorption, only certain lipid soluble substances are absorbed
- The majority of absorption occurs in the small intestine
- Small amount of fluid loss via GIT, represents only 4% of total fluid lost each day (most fluid loss is via the kidneys and respiratory system)

Basic mechanisms of absorption:

- Occurs through (1) Active transport, (2) Diffusion, (3) Solvent drag
    - Active transport; energy is used to transport the substance
    - Diffusion; a passive process via random movement
    - Solvent drag; dissolved substances dragged across with a solvent

2.2 Liver and Pancreas

Questions

1. Name the functions of the liver.
    (a) Carbohydrate, protein and lipid metabolism
    (b) Synthesis of plasma proteins
    (c) Detoxification
    (d) Immune modification

2. What is bile made of?
   Water, bile salts (highest concentration after H_2O), bilirubin, cholesterol, fatty acids, lecithin and electrolytes (Na^+, K^+, Ca^{2+}, Cl^- and HCO_3^-)

3. What is the function of bile?
   Bile is needed for the absorption of fat as well as an excretory route for lipid soluble waste products into the GIT

4. Name primary bile salts.
   Primary bile salts are cholic acid and chenodeoxycholic acid

5. Where are bile salts absorbed?
   94% are reabsorbed in the small intestine, largely in the terminal ileum.

6. Name three causes of high blood ammonia.
   High blood levels of ammonia can be due to liver dysfunction, portal hypertension with shunting or overproduction in the liver.

7. Name the exocrine enzymes released from the pancreas.
    (a) Protein digestion: Trypsin (most abundant), chymotrypsin, elastase and carboxypolypeptidases
    (b) Fat: Pancreatic lipase, cholesterol esterase and phospholipase A
    (c) Carbohydrate: Pancreatic amylase

Short notes
Liver

The liver has many functions;

- Carbohydrate, protein and lipid metabolism
- Synthesis of plasma proteins
- Detoxification
- Immune modification

Bile (500–1000 mL/day) is made up of water, bile salts/acids, bilirubin, cholesterol, fatty acid, lecithin, Na^+, K^+, Ca^{2+}, Cl^- and HCO_3^-

Bile is secreted from the liver and then stored and concentrated in the gallbladder by:

- Active absorption of Na^+ through the gallbladder epithelium
- Secondary absorption of Cl^-, water and diffusible constituents

Bile is needed for the absorption of fat as well as an excretory route for lipid soluble waste products in the GIT.

Bile salts- Made from cholesterol in liver

- The rate of synthesis in liver can be up to 0.6 g/day (normal 0.2–0.4 g/day).
- Total pool is 3.5 g
- Secretion of bile is dependent on the availability of bile salts.
- Primary bile salts are cholic acid and chenodeoxycholic acid.
- Secondary bile salts formed in colon due to bacteria - deoxycholic acid, lithocholic acid and ursodeoxycholic acid.
- They have a dual role in fat digestion:
  - Emulsify large fat particles into minute particles
  - Formation of micelles.
- Enterohepatic circulation — 94% of bile salts are reabsorbed in the small intestine.

Bile pigments (bilirubin and biliverdin): Bilirubin is formed from the breakdown of haemoglobin. It is initially unconjugated bilirubin (hydrophobic) and is conjugated in the liver with glucuronic acid to form bilirubin diglucuronide (hydrophilic). Bilirubin is converted to urobilinogen in the small intestine by bacteria.

- Jaundice is due to an excess of bilirubin in the blood from excess production, decreased uptake, impaired metabolism, or decreased secretion.

Ammonia metabolism is closely controlled due to potential CNS toxicity. Liver in the only organ that can converted ammonia to urea, which can then be excreted in the urine. Ammonia is predominately excreted from the colon and kidneys.

- High blood levels can be due to liver dysfunction, portal hypertension with shunting or overproduction in the liver.

Pancreas
Stimulation for secretion is vagal (acetylcholine) and hormonal (cholecystokinin and secretin)
Endocrine portion: (*see* Chap. 1) Insulin (β cells) and glucagon (α cells)
Exocrine portion: Enzymes produced by the pancreatic acini cells as zymogens. Trypsinogen cleaved by enterokinase to trypsin in duodenum. Trypsin activates other enzymes.

- Protein digestion – Trypsin (most abundant), chymotrypsin and carboxypolypeptidases.
- Fat – Pancreatic lipase, cholesterol esterase and phospholipase A
- Carbohydrate- Pancreatic amylase

2.3 Stomach, Small Intestine and Large Intestine

Questions

1. Which areas of the stomach are HCl and gastrin released?
   HCl is mostly released from the fundus and body. Gastrin is released from the pylorus.

2. What is released from gastric parietal cells? Chief cells?
   Parietal cells release HCl and intrinsic factor. Chief cells release pepsinogen and gastric lipase.

3. Explain the mechanism of HCl release in the stomach.
   HCl is released due to a variety of different stimuli ie vagal activity (which also stimulates chief and mucous cells), gastrin and histamine.
   Histamine is secreted by enterochromaffin-like (ECL) cells. The rate of HCl production by parietal cells is directly proportional to the activity of ECL cells. ECL cells are stimulated by gastrin production from the antral mucosa (Fig. 2.2).

4. What accounts for the largest increase in surface area of the small intestine?
   The microvilli.

5. What are the functions of the large intestine?
   Absorption of water and electrolytes, as well as storage of faeces.

6. Explain the handling of Na^+, Cl^-, HCO_3^- in the large intestine?
   Na^+ is actively absorbed and with it, Cl^- and water. The mucosa secrete HCO_3^-, helping to neutralise the acidic end products of bacterial action.

Short Notes
Stomach
Major functions of the stomach are:

1. Storage of food (up to 1.5 L)
2. Mixing of food with gastric secretions to make chyme

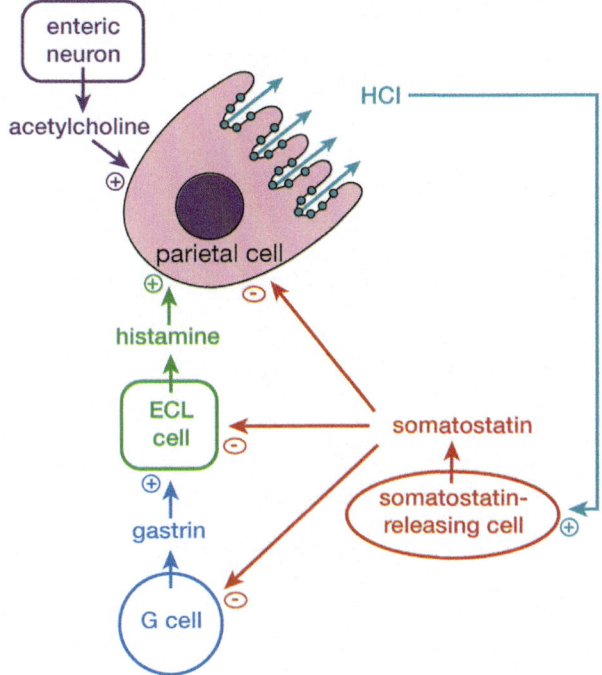

Fig. 2.2 HCl release

3. Controlled emptying of chyme into the duodenum
   (a) The pylorus is the distal opening of the stomach. Circular muscle is 50–100% greater and remains tonically contracted. Signals from the duodenum control gastric emptying.

   The stomach generally has very poor absorption, only certain lipid soluble substances pass through.

   Gastric secretion: The control of secretion from the stomach has three phases:

(a) Cephalic – secretion in response to sight, smell, taste or thought of food
(b) Gastric – secretion in response to stretching of the stomach and presence of food in the stomach
(c) Intestinal – secretion in response to the presence of chyme in the duodenum

   Mucous secreting cells line the entire stomach.
   Two types of tubular glands;

1. Oxyntic (mostly at the fundus) – HCl and pepsinogen (Fig. 2.3).
   (a) They have mucous cells at the top of the gland, then oxyntic or parietal cells (HCl and IF) and then chief cells (pepsinogen and gastric lipase).

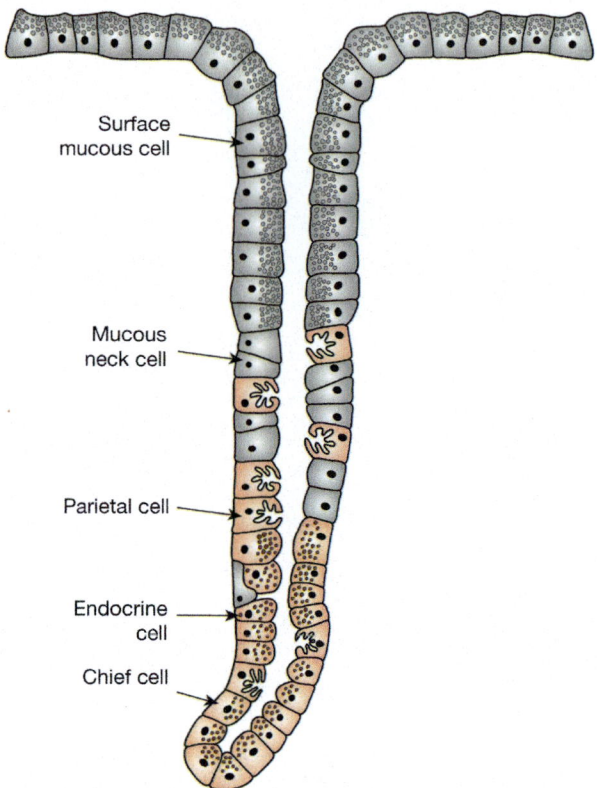

Fig. 2.3 Oxyntic gland

- HCl is released from a variety of different stimuli; vagal activity (which also stimulates chief and mucous cells), gastrin and histamine. Histamine is secreted by enterochromaffin-like (ECL) cells. The rate of HCl production from parietal cells is directly proportional to the activity of ECL cell. ECL cells are stimulated by gastrin production from the antral mucosa (Fig. 2.2).
- Pepsinogen- activated when it comes in contact with HCl. The release is due to acetylcholine from the vagus nerve and acid in the stomach.

2. Pyloric (found in the distal 20% of the stomach) – G Cells (gastrin) and mucous. Gastrin is secreted by G cells in the antrum in response to neurotransmitters, gastrin releasing peptide (GRP) or bombesin and oligopeptides in the lumen.

Small intestine
There are two types of movements in the small intestine.

1. Propulsion with peristalsis
2. Segmentation contractions

Fig. 2.4 Crypts of Lieberkuhn

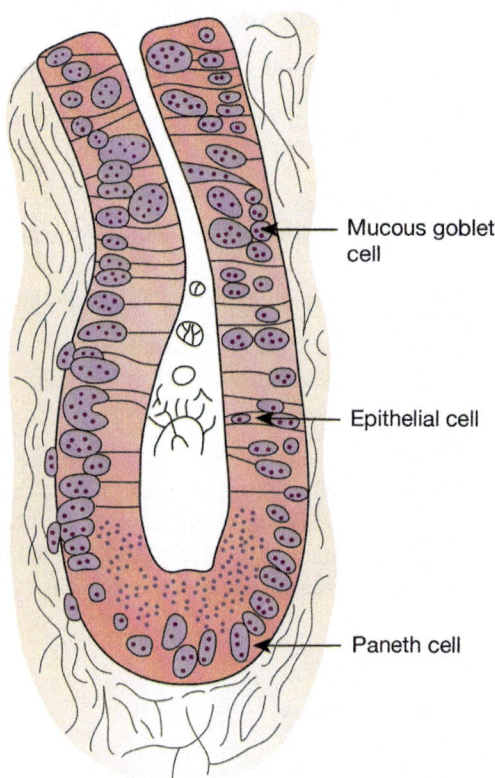

Ileocaecal valve prevents backflow from the colon into the small intestine up to a pressure of 50–60 cm H_2O.

- Surface thrown into numerous folds
    - Firstly are valvulae conniventes → project up to 8 mm → ↑ surface area by three times, especially in the duodenum and jejunum.
    - Villi located over the entire surface → project about 1 mm → ↑ surface area by ten times, fade out distally
    - On each villous is a brush border (microvilli) with each cell projecting up to 1000 nm → ↑ surface area by 20 times

In first part of SI there are large number of mucosal Brunner's glands, which secrete alkaline fluid and mucin, to help protect from acidity of chyme.

Crypts of Lieberkuhn - Contain mucous goblet cells, paneth cells, enteroendocrine cells and enterocytes (Fig. 2.4).

Enterocytes contain digestive enzymes that digest specific food substances while they are being absorbed through the epithelium (e.g. peptidases, sucrose, maltase, isomaltase and lactase and intestinal lipase).

Absorption in the Small Intestine

- Capable of absorbing significant quantities, typically;
  - 300–400 g of CHO^-, 100 g of fat, 50–100 mg of amino acids, 50–100 mg ions, 7–8 L H_2O

Large intestine

Principle functions are absorption of water and electrolytes as well as storage of faeces.

Two types of movements (slower than the small intestine):

1. Mixing movements or haustration
2. Slow propulsive movements which take 8–15 h to travel from the ileocaecal valve to the anus.

1500 mL of chyme passes through the ileocaecal valve, the large intestine absorbs the majority of this and leaves only 100–200 mL to be excreted in the faeces. Maximum absorption is 8 L. Na^+ is actively absorbed and with it Cl^- and water. The mucosa secretes HCO_3^- to help neutralise the acidic end products of bacterial action K is secreted in the large intestine.

2.4 Hormones

Questions

1. What is gastrin released in response to?
   Stomach contents and distension, vagal nerve discharge, amino acids, hypercalcaemia and tryptophan.

2. Explain how gastrin causes HCl release?
   Gastrin is transported in the *bloodstream* to the enterochromaffin-like (ECL) cells in the fundus and body of the stomach. These cells release histamine which acts on the parietal cells to cause HCl secretion.

3. Why are patients who have proximal small bowel resections at risk of peptic ulcer disease?
   This is because gastrin, secreted by G cells in the stomach antrum, is primarily inactivated in the kidney and small intestine. After a proximal small bowel resection, there is more gastrin in the bloodstream to stimulate histamine secretion. This, in turn, stimulates increased HCl secretion by parietal cells.

4. What hormone is a powerful stimulant of pancreatic enzyme secretion?
   Cholecystokinin, released by the enteroendocrine (I) cells of the small intestine.

5. List the effects of cholecystokinin release.

   (a) Acini secretion of enzyme rich pancreatic juice
   (b) Gallbladder contraction and sphincter of Oddi relaxation

(c) Trophic effect on pancreas
(d) Stimulation of hepatic bile flow

6. Which part of the pancreas does secretin act on?
This works on the pancreatic ducts to release HCO_3^- rich secretions to help neutralise the acidic chyme as it enters the duodenum.

Short notes

Gastrin:

- Released from the G cells in antrum of stomach and the first part of the duodenum
- Two forms G17 and G34
- Transported in the *bloodstream* to the enterochromaffin-like (ECL) cells. These cells release histamine, which acts on the parietal cells to release HCl.
- Released as a result of stomach distension, stomach contents, vagal nerve discharge, increased Ca^{2+} and tryptophan.
- Main action is to cause HCl and pepsin secretion
- Needed for mucosal growth

Secretin:

- Released by the S cells of the small intestine
- Released in response to acidic gastric juice and amino acids in the duodenum
- Causes HCO_3- rich pancreatic juice release from the pancreatic ducts
- Augments pancreatic secretion
- Inhibits gastric secretion and motility

Cholecystokinin:

- Released by enteroendocrine (I) cells of the small intestine
- Released due to presence of fatty acids and amino acids in the small intestine
- Causes enzyme rich secretion from the acinar cells of pancreas, relaxation of sphincter of Oddi, contraction of the gallbladder and increased hepatic bile flow.

Name	Source	Trigger	Action
Gastrin	G-cells (antral mucosa and first part of duodenum)	Stomach contents and distension, vagal discharge, amino acids, hypercalcaemia, tryptophan	Gastric acid secretion at fundus and pepsin secretion, trophic action
Cholecystokinin (CCK)	I-cells and nerves	Products of digestion (peptides, a.a. and fatty acid)	Gallbladder contraction and sphincter of Oddi relaxation, acini secretion of enzyme rich pancreatic juice, trophic effect on pancreas, stimulation of hepatic bile flow.
Secretin	S-cells	Protein digestion and acid in the upper part of the duodenum	↑ bicarbonate secretion and watery pancreatic secretions Inhibits gastric acid secretion Augments action CCK Inhibits gastric motility

Name	Source	Trigger	Action
GIP	K-cells	Glucose and fat in the duodenum	Stimulates insulin secretion
Vasoactive intestinal peptide (VIP)	Nerve endings	Fats	↑ electrolyte and H_2O secretion and relaxes intestinal smooth muscle
Motilin	Enterochromaffin cells	Potentiated by erythromycin	Contraction of smooth muscle in the stomach and intestines

2.5 Absorption of Nutrients

Questions

1. Explain the way that glucose enters the enterocytes.
   Glucose is absorbed via secondary active transport of Na^+.
   It occurs in two phases – active transport of Na^+ ions through the basolateral membrane encourages secondary active transport of glucose and Na^+ through the brush border by sodium-dependent glucose transport (SGLT, Na^+ glucose cotransporter). Once inside the cell, glucose transporter 2 (GLUT2) transports glucose out of cell into the interstitium.

2. What happens to fatty acids once they have been absorbed into the enterocytes?
   This depends on the number of carbons in the fatty acid chain. The majority are long chain FA (ie greater than 12C) and are taken up in the SER and reformed into new triglycerides and these are then released as chylomicrons into the thoracic lymphatic duct (80–90%). Short and medium FA (ie less than 12C) can be directly absorbed into the portal blood system.

3. What are micelles?
   These are small lipid molecules made up of 20–40 molecules of bile salts surrounding fatty acids and monoglycerides. They are used to ferry fatty acids and monoglycerides to the enterocyte brush border. The fatty acids and monoglycerides can then diffuse across the cell membrane. The bile salts remain in the GI lumen.

4. What is the protein requirement of adults?
   Protein requirement is 1.2–1.5 g/kg/day

5. What is the ideal pH for pepsin to work?
   pH 2.0–3.0

6. What percentage of protein is absorbed?
   >95%

7. Why does gastric acid aid the absorption of non-haem iron?
   This is because iron is absorbed in the proximal duodenum in its ferrous form (Fe^{2+}). The low pH oxides the Fe^{3+} to Fe^{2+}.

8. How long do Vitamin B12 stores last for?
   3–5 years.

9. What biochemical abnormality is seen with a gastric outlet obstruction?
   Hypochloraemic, hypokalaemic metabolic alkalosis. Loss of HCl and K^+ from the stomach.
10. Why would a patient who has had their terminal ileum (TI) resected have issues with steatorrhea?
    They have fat maldigestion. This is due to bile salt malabsorption and failure of the enterohepatic circulation, which occurs when more than 100 cm of TI has been resected

Short notes
Carbohydrates - patients require 25 kcal/kg/day.
Three major sources of carbohydrate—sucrose (glucose + fructose), lactose (glucose + galactose) and starches. Cellulose is present but cannot be readily broken down.
Digestion begins at the mouth with ptyalin (alpha-amylase) which is inactivated by stomach acid. By this stage 30–40% of the starches will have been hydrolysed. Digestion resumes in small intestine with pancreatic amylase to form maltose (2× glucose molecules) or other small glucose polymers. The enterocytes contain sucrase, lactase, maltase and alpha-dextrinase which break down oligosaccharide carbohydrates to monosaccharides. Final product of digestion is a monosaccharide. Glucose is absorbed via co-transport with the active absorption of Na^+. It occurs in two phases – active transport of Na^+ ions through the basolateral membrane. This encourages the secondary active transport of glucose through the brush border by sodium-dependent glucose transport (SGLT, Na^+ glucose cotransporter). Glucose transporter 2 (GLUT2) transports glucose out of cell into interstitium. Once out of the cells, as they are water soluble, the pass out of the enterocyte passively into the portal circulation. Galactose is transported in the same way. Fructose is transported by facilitated diffusion (Fig. 2.5).

Fat
10–15% of daily calorie intake is from fats. Largely absorbed in the upper small intestine. 95% is absorbed in adults. 85–90% in children.
The largest dietary source of fats is neutral fats known as triglycerides (glycerol and 3× fatty acids side chains). There is also a small amount of phospholipids, cholesterol and cholesterol esters.
Digestion starts in the mouth with a small amount of lingual lipase. Small amount in stomach from gastric lipase.
In the small intestine, it needs to have been emulsified by bile salts and lecithin. This is needed as the lipase enzymes are water soluble, therefore, can only act on fat globules on their surface.
TGs are mainly digested by pancreatic lipase, plus a small amount of enteric lipase. Digested to fatty acid and 2-monoglycerides. Cholesterol by cholesterol ester hydrolase and phospholipids are digested by phospholipase A2.
Then they form micelles – (3–6 nm) 20–40 molecules of bile salt with fatty acid and monoglyceride center. Micelles ferry fatty acids and monoglycerides to the brush border where they can be absorbed. At the brush border the monoglycerides and fatty acids diffuse immediately out of the micelles and into the interior

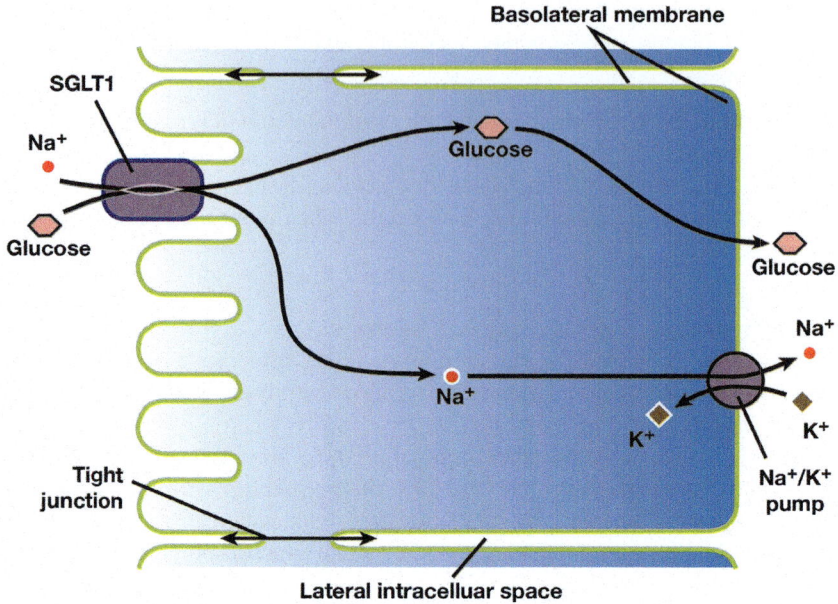

Fig. 2.5 Glucose absorption

of the enterocyte. This process leaves the bile salts in the chyme. In the absence of bile salts only 50% of fat is absorbed.

After entering the epithelial cell, the fatty acids and monoglycerides are taken up in the SER and formed into new TGs and released as chylomicrons into the thoracic lymphatic duct (80–90%). Short and medium chain FA (ie less than 12C) can be directly absorbed into the portal blood system.

Short chain fatty acids – 60% acetate, 25% propionate, 15% butyrate, formed by colonic bacteria, contribute a significant amount to total caloric intake.

Protein

Protein requirement is 1.2–1.5 g/kg/day.

>95% of protein is digested and absorbed.

Protein digestion begins in the stomach with pepsin (most active at pH 2–3). The majority of protein digestion occurs in the upper small intestine. The enzymes are trypsin, chymotrypsin, carboxypolypeptidase and elastase. Most proteins are absorbed as di- and tripeptides. Microvilli on enterocytes contain peptidases - aminopolypeptidases and dipeptidases. The di- and tri-peptidases are then digested to singular amino acids in the cells and pass into the bloodstream. The energy for the absorption comes from the sodium transport-mechanism explained above.

At least seven different transport systems exist. Absorption is rapid in duodenum and jejunum. 50% from ingested food, 25% from proteins in digestive juice and 25% from desquamated mucosal cells. Infants can absorb whole protein from the intestinal tract, adults require digestion.

Iron

In health the rate of iron loss from the body is small (0.6 mg/day in men). Iron stores are regulated by absorption. Males need 0.5–1 mg/day but ingest around 20 mg, hence only a small percentage of what is ingested is absorbed. Absorption is controlled by recent dietary intake, iron stores and state of erythropoiesis.

Most dietary iron is in its ferric form Fe^{3+} but needs to be Fe^{2+} for absorption. Absorption of non-haem iron is increased by acid in the stomach and vitamin C. It is inhibited by the presence of HCO_3^- in the duodenum and phytic acid in cereal products.

Absorption occurs predominantly in the duodenum.

Transport of Fe^{2+} into enterocytes occurs via divalent metal transporter 1 (DMT1). Some is stored as ferritin inside the enterocyte. The remainder is transported from the basolateral membrane by ferroportin 1. In the plasma it is converted to Fe^{3+} and transported by transferrin.

70% of iron is in haemoglobin, 3% in myoglobin and the rest is in ferritin form.

B12 – water soluble vitamin which acts as a co-enzyme in DNA and RBC synthesis.

Absorption requires intrinsic factor, released by parietal cells in the gastric fundus and body. IF binds with B12 in the small intestine and, along with trypsin, facilitates efficient absorption of B12 in the terminal ileu.

- Sodium

    5–8 g ingested, 30 g secreted → 25–35 g absorbed (1/7th of total body Na^+)

    - Mechanism; Secondary active transport → Na^+ pumped out, concentration gradient formed → Na^+ enters from chyme
    - NOTE: H_2O is absorbed into the paracellular spaces concurrently
    - NOTE: Na^+ plays an important role in the absorption of sugars and a.a.
    - NOTE: Aldosterone greatly enhances Na^+ absorption (and therefore water)

- Chloride

    - Rapid process occurring mainly by diffusion (follows Na^+ ions)

- Bicarbonate ions

    - Large amounts are secreted in the pancreatic and biliary secretions
    - Indirect mechanism; H^+ secreted → forms carbonic acid → dissociates into CO_2 and H_2O → CO_2 is absorbed and expired in the lungs (same mechanism as the kidneys)
    - NOTE: Ileum and LI actively secrete bicarbonate ions (in exchange for Cl^-) to neutralize acid products from bacteria

- Potassium, Magnesium and phosphate are all actively absorbed

    - Monovalent ions are easily absorbed while bivalent ions are much slower

2.6 Disorders of Swallowing and of the Oesophagus

Questions

1. What is the biochemical consequence of vomiting caused by pyloric stenosis?
   Hypochloremic metabolic alkalosis
2. Which parts of the esophagus are normally closed?
   It is normally closed at both ends (cricopharyngeus proximally and lower esophageal sphnicter (LES) distally)
3. What is achalasia?
   It is a disorder characterised by ineffective esophageal parastalsis and ineffectual lower esophageal relaxation.
4. Explain the pathophysiology of pernicious anaemia.
   Pernicious anaemia in gastric atrophy is due to a failure of normal secretion of intrinsic factor (required for B12 absorption). In the absence of intrinsic factor, 0.02% of vitamin B12 is absorbed → failed maturation of red blood cells.

Short notes

- Paralysis of the swallowing mechanism

  - May occur with damage to CrN 5,9,10, poliomyelitis, encephalitis, muscular dystrophy
  - Abnormalities include;

    Complete abrogation of the swallowing act
    Failure of the glottis to close → aspiration
    Failure of the soft palate and uvula to close → food passes into the nose

- Achalasia and Mega-oesophagus

  - Lower oesophageal sphincter fails to relax → food passage is impeded

    Unclear aetiology, may be due to damage to the neural network of the myenteric plexus in the lower 2/3 of oesophagus
    This may cause significant distension of the oesophagus (1L or more) which can lead to infection, ulceration or malignancy (SCC)
    Balloon dilation, antispasmodics, Botox and surgery may be useful treatment

Disorders of the Stomach

- Gastritis (inflammation of the gastric mucosa)

  - May be chronic (superficial or causing almost complete atrophy) or acute (with ulceration)
  - Normal gastric barrier/protection from

    Highly resistant mucous cells with a viscid and adherent mucous
    Tight junctions between epithelial cells
    Allows for a 1:100,000 H+ concentration gradient
    In gastritis the permeability is greatly increased

2 Gastrointestinal Physiology

- Gastric Atrophy
  - With chronic gastritis and autoimmunity → gastric atrophy → pernicious anaemia and achlorhydria
  - Achlorhydria (failure to secrete HCl → pH unable to <6.5)

    Results in pepsin not being secreted or activated
    Clinically other enzymes take over with little consequence

  - Pernicious anaemia in gastric atrophy

    Normal secretion includes intrinsic factor (required for B12 absorption)

    In the absence of intrinsic factor, 0.02% of vitamin B12 is absorbed → failed maturation of red blood cells

    Also occurs with gastrectomy or terminal ileectomy

- Peptic ulcer
  - Excoriated area most often seen at cardia, pylorus and most frequently the first few cm of duodenum
  - Due to imbalance between secretion of acid/juice and protection
  - There are many normal protective mechanisms to help stop this happening, but may occur due to

    Excess secretion of acid and pepsin by the gastric mucosa
    Diminished ability of the gastroduodenal mucosa barrier to protect

  - Specific causes

    H. pylori (75% of those with peptic ulceration)
    Aspirin/NSAID (inhibit mucous production), smoking, alcohol

Disorders of the small intestine

- Pancreatic failure from inflammation, blockage, or resection
  - Results in as much as 60% of fat being malabsorbed
- Malabsorption of the small intestine mucosa (sprue)
  - Non-tropical (a.k.a. idiopathic, coeliac, gluten enteropathy)

    Destruction of microvilli/villi leading to malabsorption

  - Tropical

    Exact infectious cause, often responds to antibiotics

  - Often starts as steatorrhoea, and may progress to protein, carbohydrate and electrolyte malabsorption
  - Results in severe nutritional deficiency, osteomalacia, poor blood coagulation and macrocytic anaemia

Disorders of the large intestine

- Constipation
  - May be secondary to megacolon from aganglionic or poorly ganglionic segments
- Diarrhoea
  - Enteritis
  - Cholera
  - Psychogenic
  - Inflammatory Bowel Disease (Ulcerative colitis, Crohn's Colitis)
- Paralysis in spinal cord injuries – loss of normal bowel function, may be assisted by enemas

General Disorders

- Vomiting
  - Begins with antiperistalsis → pushed up contents → excites upper small intestine → initiates the vomiting act
  - Vomiting act → deep breath → raising of the hyoid and larynx → closing of the glottis/lifting of the soft palate
  - Chemoceptor trigger zone may be stimulated by drugs or motion sickness
  - Nausea part of vomiting prodrome
- Bowel obstruction
  - Blockage site influences nature of situation

    Pyloric → stomach contents
    High small intestine → Lots of liquid and bile
    Low small intestine → Lots of basic fluid → acidosis and faecal character
    Note that the distension usually stimulates secretion, which in the case of a bowel obstruction can lead to dehydration
    LI obstruction usually does not cause vomiting in the first instance, usually there is constipation which may later be followed by vomiting

Chapter 3
Cardiovascular Physiology

S. Ali Mirjalili, Lucy Hinton, and Kevin Ellyett

3.1 The Cardiac Cycle: Mechanical Events

Questions

1. What causes the first heart sound?
   The closure of the atrioventricular valves - mitral and tricuspid.
   This indicates the beginning of systole and the start of isovolumetric contraction.

2. What percentage of ventricular filling does atrial contraction contribute to?
   25–30%.

3. What are normal values for end diastolic volume (EDV) and end systolic volume (ESV)?
   EDV- *volume in the ventricle at the end of diastole* = 130 mL.
   ESV- *volume remaining in the ventricle at the end of systole* = 60 mL.

4. How is the stroke volume (SV) calculated?
   SV is the amount of blood pumped out of the ventricle in one contraction. This is calculated by;
   SV = EDV − ESV.
   SV = 130 mL − 60 mL.
   The stroke volume is 70 mL.

S. A. Mirjalili (✉)
Department of Anatomy and Medical Imaging, University of Auckland, Auckland, New Zealand
e-mail: a.mirjalili@auckland.ac.nz

L. Hinton
Department of General Surgery, Tauranga Hospital, Tauranga, New Zealand

K. Ellyett
University of Auckland, Auckland, New Zealand

Auckland Hospital, Auckland, New Zealand

© Springer Nature Singapore Pte Ltd. and People's Medical Publishing House Co. Ltd. 2019
S. A. Mirjalili (ed.), *Physiology for General Surgical Sciences Examination (GSSE)*, https://doi.org/10.1007/978-981-13-2580-9_3

5. How do you calculate the ejection fraction?
   This is the percentage of blood that is ejected from the ventricle each cardiac cycle. This is calculated by;
   EF = SV/EDV.
   EF = 70 mL/130 mL
   It is normally ~60–65%.

6. Are the third and fourth heart sounds always pathological?
   No, the third heart sound can be physiological in children, athletes and pregnant women. However, the fourth heart sound is pathological.

7. During exercise, which part of the heart cycle reduces the most (systole or diastole)? What effect does this have on coronary artery filling?
   Proportionally diastole decreases more.
   This means that there is less time for left coronary artery filling as this occurs most rapidly throughout diastole.

8. Please label the diagram of the JVP wave and explain what the different parts represent.

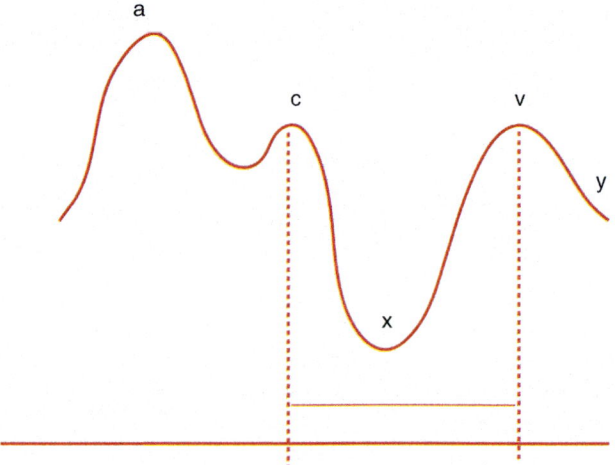

- 'a' ↑ pressure during atrial systole and contraction
- 'c' ↑ in atrial pressure as ventricular systole begins
- 'x descent' following ventricular stretching and atrial relaxation
- 'v' wave is from ↑ in Rt atrial pressure just before AV valves open caused by atrial filling
- 'y descent' following the valves opening

9. Which ventricle ejects blood first (the right or the left)
   The right ventricle. This is because the pulmonary circulation is a lower pressure system than the systemic circulation so the pulmonary valve opens before the aortic valve.

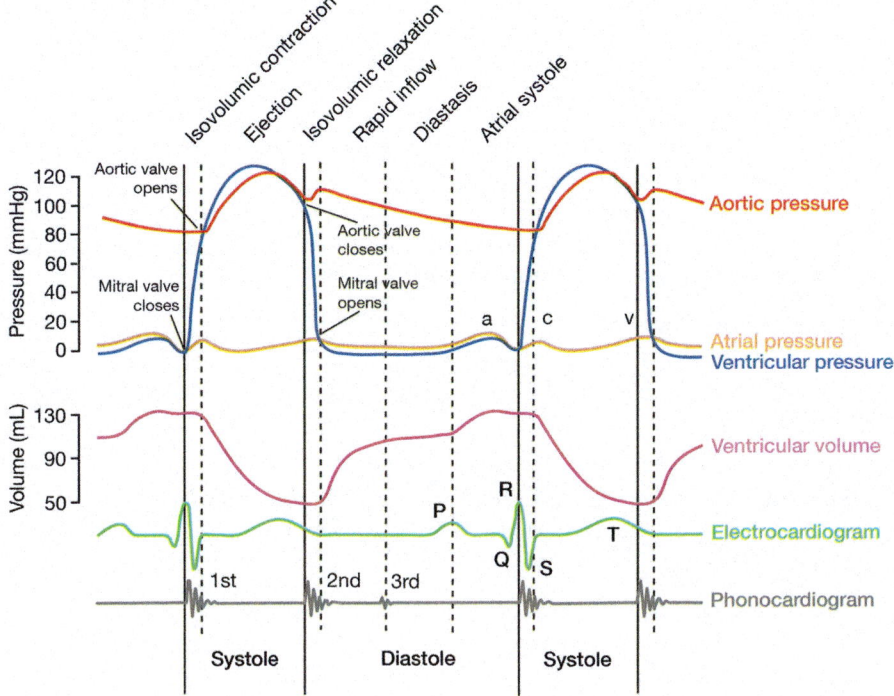

Fig. 3.1 Cardiac cycle

Cardiac cycle (Fig. 3.1)
Timing
The cardiac cycle is divided into systole and diastole.

- At a heart rate (HR) of 75 bpm, the cardiac cycle lasts 800 ms^{-1}. This is divided into 1/3 systole (270 ms^{-1}) and 2/3 diastole (530 ms^{-1})
- In severe exercise the HR can increase to 200 bpm, the cardiac cycle therefore decreases to 300 ms^{-1}. This is now divided into ~160 ms^{-1} for systole and 140 ms^{-1} for diastole (proportionally greater decrease in diastole)

Ventricular systole
Two components;
(1) Isovolumetric contraction and (2) Ventricular ejection.

1. Isovolumetric contraction:
   When ventricular pressure exceeds atrial pressure the atrioventricular valves close (first heart sound) indicating the start of systole → Ventricular depolarization causes ventricular muscle contraction, both the mitral and aortic valves are shut, so contraction causes the ventricular size to decrease, but there is no

movement of blood, so the intra-ventricular pressure rises. *This is the greatest pressure rise in the cardiac cycle.* This causes the 'c' wave on the JVP waveform as the tricuspid valve bulges into the right atrium.

2. Ventricular ejection:
   When the pressure inside the ventricle exceeds the aortic pressure, the aortic valve opens. Blood is ejected rapidly, then more slowly, as the muscle loses tension → When the pressure inside the aorta exceeds the pressure in the ventricle the aortic valve closes (second heart sound). At this stage the ventricles contain around 60 mL of blood (end systolic volume, ESV)

Ventricular diastole
Four components;
(1) Isovolumetric relaxation and (2) Rapid inflow (3) Diastasis (4) Atrial contraction;

1. Isovolumetric relaxation:
   When the aortic value shuts at the end of systole, then ventricular muscle relaxes, but there is no movement of blood as both valves are shut, so the intra-ventricular pressure decreases.
2. Rapid inflow:
   When the pressure in the ventricle falls below the atrial pressure, the atrioventricular valves open. The ventricular filling is initially rapid.
3. Diastasis:
   The filling then slows as the pressure inside the ventricle increases.
4. Atrial systole:
   Contraction of the atria near the end of diastole drives 25–30% more blood into the ventricles. Some blood regurgitates back into the vessels, which is seen as the 'a' wave of the JVP wave.
   Ventricles contain around 130 mL of blood at this stage (end diastolic volume, EDV)

Heart sounds

First HS: Closure of atrioventricular valves (mitral and tricuspid). Indicates the start of systole.
Second HS: Closure of aortic and pulmonary valves. Indicates the start of diastole.
Third HS: Oscillation of blood between the walls of the ventricles caused by the inflow of blood from the atria. Heard at the beginning of the middle third of diastole. Normal in youth, athletes and pregnant women. If heard in adults, it may indicate heart failure.
Fourth HS: Contraction of the atria in late diastole pushing blood into a stiff or hypertrophic ventricle. Always pathological.

3 Cardiovascular Physiology

Pressures, Ventricular Volume, Heart Sounds and the ECG (Fig. 3.1)

	Late diastole	Isovolumetric C	Ejection	Isovolumetric R	Diastole
Pressure (aorta)	85–80 (falling)	Drop to diastolic	↑ rapidly	Dicrotic notch	Gradual ↓
Pressure (vent)	↑ slightly	↑ sharply	Slows & then starts to ↓	↓ rapidly	Minimal
Pressure (atrium)	↑ w/contraction	c-wave from ventricular bulging	Gradually ↑	Continues to ↑	Minimal
Volume (vent)	Topped up to EDV	No change	Rapidly then gradually ↓	No change	Plateaus
Heart sounds	4th	1st		2nd	3rd
ECG	P wave	QRS	1st part of T	2nd part of T	Nil

JVP (Fig. 3.2)

- RA communicates with JVP and transmits waves
    - 'a' ↑ pressure during atrial systole and contraction
    - 'c' ↑ in atrial pressure as ventricular systole begins
    - 'x descent' following ventricular stretching and atrial relaxation

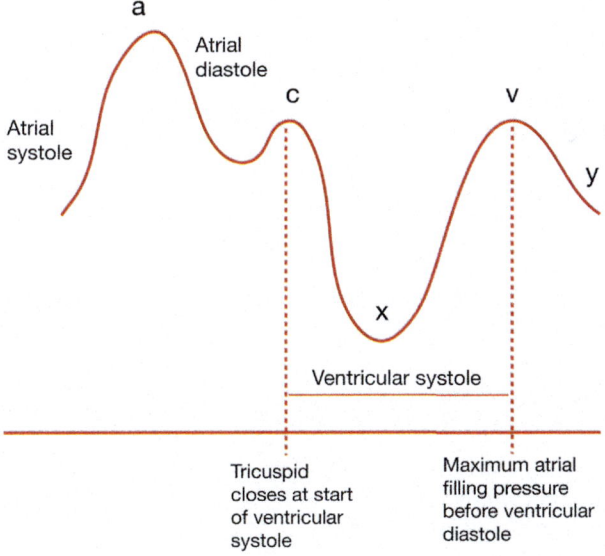

Fig. 3.2 JVP wave

- 'v' wave is from ↑ in Rt atrial pressure just before AV valves open caused by atrial filling
- 'y descent' following the valves opening

Asynchrony of the Right and Left Heart

- Right atrial systole and contraction begins before the left atria
- Tension in the left ventricle rises before the right ventricle, but due to lower pressures system of the pulmonary circulation, the right ventricle begins ejecting blood before the left ventricle
- Right ventricle ejects blood for longer than the left ventricle, hence the pulmonary valve closes later

Stroke Volume and Ejection Fraction

- The *stroke volume* is the amount of blood ejected from the ventricle during systole. It is calculated by end diastolic volume − end systolic volume (EDV − ESV). It is normally around 70 mL.
- The *ejection fraction* is the percentage of blood ejected from the heart each cardiac cycle. It is calculated as the stroke volume divided by end diastolic volume (SV/EDV) → normally about 60–65%

Bruit and Murmurs

- A bruit is heard over a vessel (from turbulent flow) whereas a murmur is generally over a valve
    - Stenosis of aortic/pulmonary valves and atrioventricular incompetence → systolic murmur
    - Atrioventricular stenosis and pulmonary/aortic incompetence → diastolic murmurs

3.2 Conduction with ECG

Questions

1. List some features of cardiac muscle cells.
    (a) Striated muscle
    (b) Form a syncytium
    (c) Connected by intercalated discs
    (d) Gap junctions that allow the action potential to propagate from cell to cell
    (e) T tubules

2. What fuel sources do the cardiac muscle cells use?
   They predominately use fatty acids. At rest, 60% fatty acid, 35% carbohydrate and 5% ketones and amino acids.

3. What is the resting membrane potential (RMP) of the cardiac muscle cell? Sinoatrial (SA) node?
   The cardiac muscle cells have a lower RMP than in the conducting system e.g. SA node. The RMP in the cardiac muscle cells is −90 mV in comparison with −60 mV in the SA node.

4. Describe the changes in the membrane permeability to ions during the different phase of the cardiac action potential in cardiac muscle cells.
   (a) Phase 0- Initial depolarisation due to rapid ↑ in Na^+ permeability
   (b) Phase 1- Initial repolarisation is due to inactivation of fast Na channels and outward flow of K^+ ions
   (c) Phase 2- Inward current due to influx of Ca^{2+} → plateau phase
   (d) Phase 3- Inactivation of slow Ca^{2+} channels hence there is unopposed outward flow of K^+ ions → repolarisation
   (e) Phase 4- Restoration to the RMP. Cell membrane is most permeable to K^+

5. Which part of the electrical conduction system of the heart transmits at the fastest speed?
   The Purkinje fibres, 4 ms^{-1}. See table in notes.

6. How does the parasympathetic nervous system (PSNS) act to slow the heart rate?
   It acts on the SA node. The acetylcholine (Ach) binds to muscarinic (M2) receptors and via G-proteins opens K^+ channels. This causes further movement of K^+ out of the cell and therefore hyperpolarizes it. This means it is harder for the SA node to reach threshold potential and the heart rate is slowed.

7. How do you calculate the QTc and what part of the cardiac electrical cycle does this represent?
   The QT interval corresponds to electrical systole. The QT length is inversely proportional to the HR (Fig. 3.3).

8. What does this rhythm strip show? (Fig. 3.4)
   This saw-tooth pattern is atrial flutter with a 2:1 block. This is a supraventricular tachycardia with a regular rhythm. This is due to a re-entrant circuit in the right atrium. The atrial rate in atrial flutter is usually 300 bpm (200–400 bpm) however not all of these atrial beats are conducted through to the ventricle hence there is some sort of atrioventricular (AV) block – most commonly 2:1.

Fig. 3.3 QTc
$$QTc = \frac{QT}{\sqrt{RR}}$$

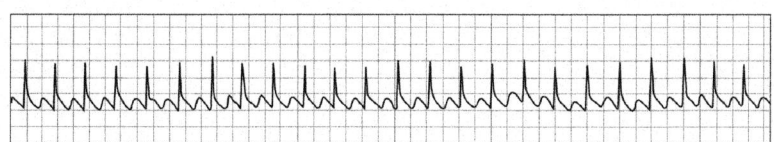

Fig. 3.4 Atrial flutter

9. What ECG changes are seen in hypokalaemia and hyperkalaemia?

    (a) Hypokalemia causes prolongation of the PR interval, U waves, T wave inversion/flattening and ST segment depression

    - Due to prolonged ventricular repolarisation
    - Later you may see prolonged segments

    (b) Hyperkalemia may get peaked T waves, prolonged PR and QRS intervals

10. How does digoxin work? What are some ECG changes seen in digoxin toxicity? Its primary mechanism is to inhibit the Na/K ATPase in the myocardium. In toxicity ECG changes include T wave inversion or biphasic T waves.

Cardiac Muscle

- Striated cells, branching to form a network or syncytium
- They make end-to-end connections through intercalated discs
- They have gap junctions between the cells to allow for action potential propagation
- T-tubules are more numerous and larger than skeletal muscle (Fig. 3.5)

Cardiac Muscle metabolism

- Many mitochondria → predominantly aerobic metabolism utilising multiple fuel sources (whatever is available)

    – At rest (60% lipid, 35% carbohydrate, 5% ketones and amino acid.)

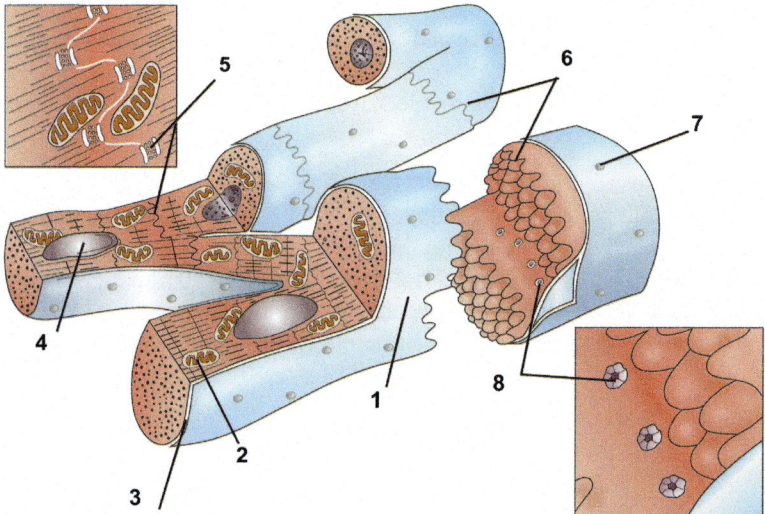

Fig. 3.5 Cardiac muscle cell

Cardiac myocyte action potential

- RMP (−90 mV) is due to outward movement of K^+ ions from the cell balanced by a small influx of Na^+ ions (Fig. 3.6)
- The action potential of cardiac muscle cells lasts longer (250 ms^{-1}) than nerve or skeletal muscle (2–4 ms^{-1}) due to a prolonged plateau phase

  - Phase 0- When threshold of −70 mV is reached, rapid depolarization occurs due to opening of voltage-gated Na^+ channels
  - Phase 1- Initial depolarization is due to inactivation of voltage-gated Na^+ channels and unopposed K^+ efflux
  - Phase 2- Inward current of Ca^{2+} due activation of L-type calcium channels → plateau phase as the K^+ efflux is matched the Ca^{2+} influx
  - Phase 3- Inactivation of slow Ca^{2+} channels → repolarisation caused by K^+ efflux
  - Phase 4- Restoration to the RMP

- Muscle contraction begins just after Phase 1 and lasts longer

  - Refractory periods – Absolute refraction (no contraction possible) followed by relative refraction (contraction under certain circumstances) → prevents tetanus

Origin and spread of cardiac activity

Location	SA node	Three atrial internodal pathways	AV node	Bundle of His	Purkinje fibres
Natural rate d/c	70–80 min^{-1}		40–60 min^{-1}		15–40 min^{-1}
Depolarisation	0.05 ms^{-1}	1 ms^{-1}	0.05 ms^{-1}	1 ms^{-1}	4 ms^{-1}

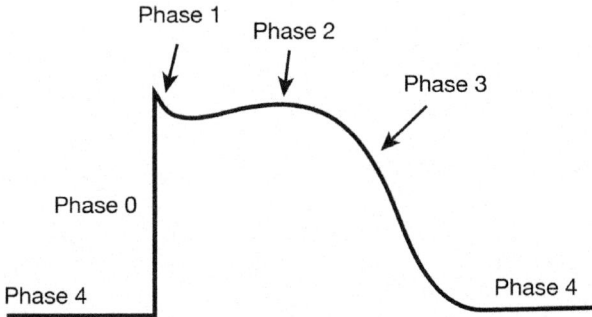

Fig. 3.6 Cardiac myocyte action potential

Electrical activity of the SA node (see Fig. 3.7)

- The electrical activity in the conducting system of the heart differs to that of the myocytes

Sinoatrial node action potential:

- Phase 4 - RMP reaches a maximum of −55 mV to −60 mV, which slowly drifts up to −40 → pre-potential
    - This is due to the 'leaky' membrane of Na. (High extracellular Na and open Na channels allow inward movement of Na). This then triggers the opening of T-type (transient) Ca channels
- Phase 0- At −40 mV, the L-type Ca channels open and cause depolarisation.
- Phase 3- L-type Ca channels inactivate within 100–150 ms^{-1} and K channels open, which causes re-polarisation.

AV node

This is the gateway of conduction between the atria and the ventricles, as otherwise the atria and ventricles are separated by the fibrous skeleton of the heart.

Control of cardiac electrical activity

- Parasympathetic nervous system- Cholinergic nerves act on the SA node causing tonic inhibition as well as decreasing excitability of the AV junctional fibres between atrial musculature and AV node, slowing transmission.
    - ACh → Muscarinic (M2) receptors → G protein → open K channels → hyperpolarization of the membrane therefore longer to reach threshold potential.
- Sympathetic nervous system- Noradrenergic fibres act on the SA node to ↑ HR and ↑ rate of conduction through AV node as well as ↑ force of contraction.
    - NA → B1 receptors → ↑ in cAMP → increased sarcolemma permeability to Na$^+$ and Ca^{2+} channels

Threshold is reached quicker

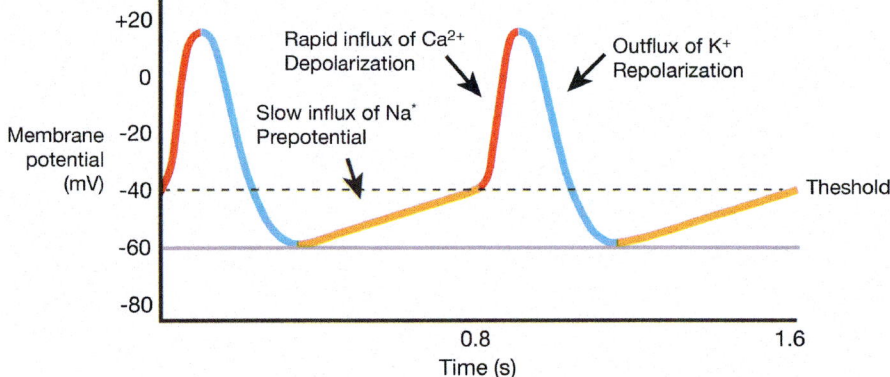

Fig. 3.7 Sinoatrial node action potential

3 Cardiovascular Physiology

ECG (Fig. 3.8)

- Paper moves at 25 mm s^{-1}
- P wave (<0.08 s) = atrial depolarization
- QRS (0.08–0.10 s) = ventricular depolarization
- T wave (0.16 s) = ventricular repolarisation
- PR interval (0.12–0.2 s) = beginning of P wave to the beginning of QRS complex
- QT interval (0.35 s) = electrical systole
    - QTc 'corrected QT interval' – QT interval is inversely proportional to HR
    - QTc = QT interval/square root of the RR interval
    - Prolonged by genetic conditions, certain drugs and metabolic conditions and predisposes to tachyarrhymias. At increased risk of developing *torsades de pointes*
- Standard bipolar limb leads record differences between LA/RA (lead I), LL/RA (lead II), LL and LA (lead III)
- Augmented limb leads, aVR, aVL and aVF record differences between RA, LA and LL
- Chest leads (V1–V6) look at the activity of the heart in a horizontal plane

Arrhythmias (Fig. 3.9)
Sinus:

- Sinus tachycardia is caused by fever, sympathetic stimulation and toxic conditions.
- Sinus bradycardia is caused by abnormal vagal activity, sick sinus syndrome and athletes.
- Sinus arrhythmia – Normal variation takes place with breathing (stretch receptors altering vagal tone)
    - Increased HR with inspiration

Extrasystoles:
Atrial ectopic foci can cause extrasystoles and abnormal p waves

- Repetitive discharge of an ectopic focus with re-entry can produce paroxysmal atrial tachycardia and atrial flutter

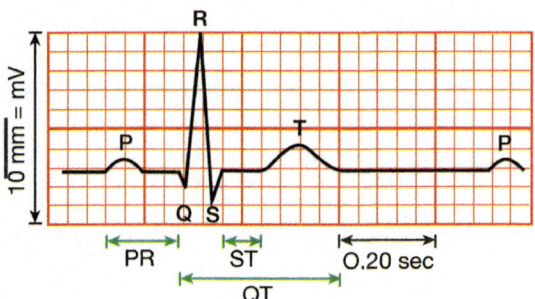

Fig. 3.8 ECG

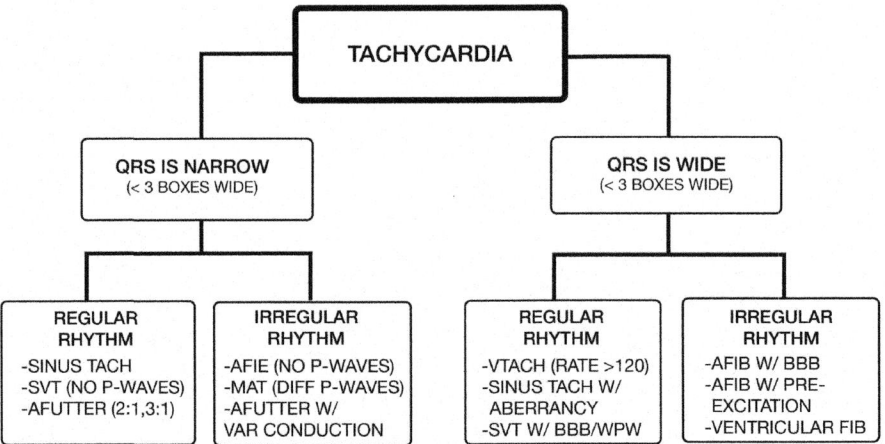

Fig. 3.9 Tachy-arrhythmias

- AV nodal or AV bundle premature contractions.

  Ventricular extrasystoles are wide and abnormally shaped QRS complexes
  Tachyarhythmias:

- AF (atrial rate 300–500 bpm) with an irregular ventricular rhythm (80–160) → ineffective and uncoordinated muscular contraction. Lose their atrial 'kick' of atrial blood into the ventricle.
- Atrial flutter (atrial rate is usually 300 bpm (200–350 bpm)), with a 2, 3 or 4 block to ventricular depolarization. The ventricular rate is therefore regular.
- Ventricular arrhythmias are wide complex

  – Paroxysmal ventricular tachycardia is due to circus movements and may result in VF
  – VF appears to be from multiple sights or re-entry, if persists from more than a few minutes is fatal

Heart Block:
May be partial (incomplete, 1′) intermittent (2′), or complete (3′)

- First-Degree Block – prolonged PR interval. Delay of conduction from atria to ventricle.
- Second-Degree Block

  – Type 1 – (Wenckebach) Progressive prolongation of the PR interval with an eventual dropping of the ventricular beat.
  – Type 2 – Intermittent non-conducted P wave, usually associated with a fixed number of non-conducted P waves to conducted P waves.

- Third-Degree Block- complete dissociation between the atria and the ventricles.

AV nodal tachycardias:

- Wolf-Parkinson-White (WPW) is due to a congenital accessory pathway. It is characterized by short PR, prolonged QRS and *Delta* wave (slurred up stroke of the QRS complex due to abnormal conduction between A + V). This abnormal movement is usually initiated by an abnormal beat e.g. premature atrial contraction.

Changes in Extracellular Ions

- Hypokalemia causes prolongation of the PR interval, U waves, T wave inversion/flattening and ST segment depression
    - Due to prolonged ventricular repolarisation
    - Later you may see prolonged segments
- Hyperkalemia may get peaked T waves, flattening of P waves, prolonged PR and QRS intervals
- Hypercalcemia theoretically may stop the heart in systole – but clinically is seldom a problem
- Hypocalcemia causes ST prolongation

3.3   Cardiac Output

Questions

1. Please calculate the cardiac output in the following scenario; The CaO_2 = 0.2 mL/mL and CvO_2 0.15 mLO_2/mL blood. The VO_2 is 250 mL O_2/min.
   VO_2 = rate of oxygen consumption, CaO_2 = arterial concentration of oxygen, CvO_2 = venous concentration of oxygen
   Fick's principle = Amount of substance taken up per unit time
   (Rate of oxygen consumption)/(CaO_2 – CvO_2)
   CO = 250/(0.2 – 0.15)
   CO = 250/0.05
   CO = 5000 mL/min

2. What three factors determine the stroke volume?

   (a) Degree of filling of the ventricle, or "*preload*"
   (b) *Contractility* of the myocardium
   (c) Resistance against which the ventricle has to work, or "*afterload*".

3. Why does increasing the venous return, increase the cardiac output.
   This is because of the Frank-Starling mechanism (Fig. 3.10). Increased venous return increases the end diastolic volume (EDV) → This in turn increases the pre-contraction length of the myocytes. This results in more optimal alignment of the actin and myosin filaments and therefore a stronger contraction and greater stroke volume.

4. Name some negative inotropic agents.
   A negative inotrope is any agent that decreases the contractility of the heart. The most important physiological factor is the PSNS. Other pathological conditions such as hypoxia, hypercapnia, acidosis have negative inotrophic effects on the heart. Pharmaceutical agents such B-blockers, Ca^{2+} blockers, barbiturates and many anaesthetics.

5. At rest, what percentage of oxygen is extracted from the coronary circulation?
   ~70%. This means that the increase oxygen needed during exercise is met with increasing blood flow, controlled by local factors, namely hypoxia.

6. Name the four categories of shock.
   (a) Hypovolemic
   (b) Distributive
   (c) Cardiogenic
   (d) Obstructive

Cardiac Output

$$\text{Cardiac output}(CO) = \text{volume of blood ejected by each ventricle per minute}(SV \times HR)(\text{around } 5000\,mL/\min).$$

Measurement of Cardiac Output:

- Fick's principle:
  - Cardiac output = Amount of the substance taken up per unit time $(VO_2)/(\text{Conc } O_{2\,arterial} - \text{Conc } O_{2\,venous})$

Stroke volume depends on:

1. Degree of filling of the ventricle, or "preload"
2. Contractility of the myocardium
3. Resistance against which the ventricle has to work, or "afterload".

1. Preload
   Defined by the 'Frank-Starling mechanism'
   (a) If ↑ in venous return → ↑ in ventricular filling → ↑ in pre-contraction length → ↑ contraction → ↑ SV
   (b) Thought to result from more optimal alignment of actin and myosin filaments, and ↑ sensitivity to Ca^{2+}
   (c) Note that beyond an optimal point, stroke volume diminishes (Fig. 3.10).

2. Myocardial contractility
   (a) This refers to the intrinsic ability of the cardiac muscle fibres to contract and is independent of the degree of preload and afterload. Known as the 'inotropy'

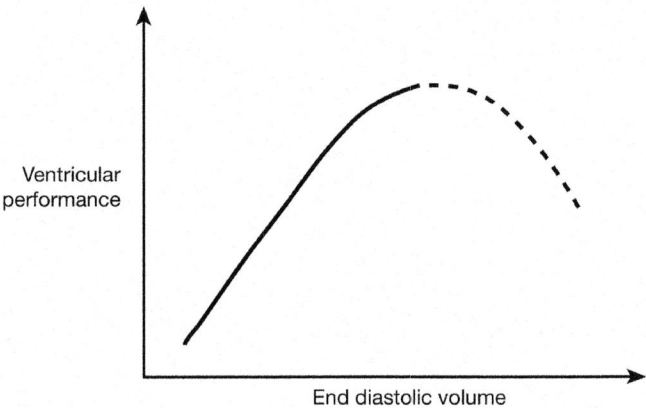

Fig. 3.10 Frank-Starling mechanism

(b) Positive inotropic agents

- Sympathetic discharge and circulating catecholamines → ↑ contractility
- B-receptors → G-proteins → adenylate cyclase → cAMP → ↑ in Ca2+ influx → enhanced cross bridges → ↑ contractile force → ↑ SV
- Also, an ↑ in HR → ↑ in free intracellular Ca^{2+} → positive inotropic effect
- Caffeine, theophylline inhibit breakdown of cAMP → positive inotropic effect
- Glucagon ↑ formation of cAMP → positive inotropic effect
- Digitalis inhibits NaK ATPase → ↑ Ca^{2+} concentration → positive inotropic effect

(c) Negative inotropic agents

- Parasympathetic → ↑ ACh → ↓ atrial contractility
- Hypercapnia, hypoxia, acidosis and heart failure → negative inotropic effect
- B-blockers, Ca^{2+} blockers, barbiturates and many anaesthetics → negative inotropic effect (Fig. 3.11)

3. Afterload
In order for the ventricle to contract needs to overcome;

(a) The tension in the ventricular wall itself
(b) The resistance offered to the ejection of blood from the AV and aorta.

In health, afterload is determined predominantly by vascular tone.

Heart rate
The sinoatrial node (intrinsic pacemaker @ 100bpm)

- +ve chronotrophic – ANS via adrenergic receptors, directly or via adrenal glands.
- −ve chronotrophic – PSNS, via the vagus nerve.

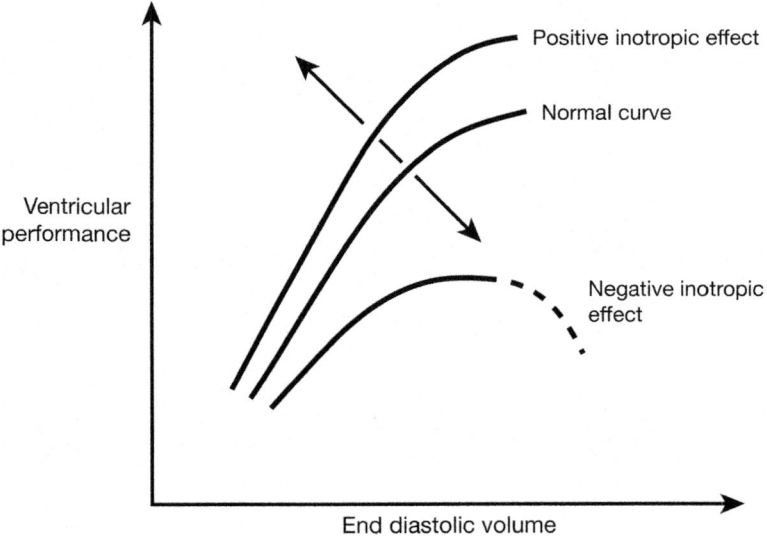

Fig. 3.11 Effect of contractility on ventricular performance

Cardiac oxygen consumption

- In a normal beating heart at rest this is 7–10 mL/100 g/min and in vigorous exercise this is 40 mL/100 g/min
- This ↑ in demand has to be met with an ↑ in supply by ↑ BF

Cycle of heart failure
Decrease CO, therefore a higher EDV with a higher RA pressure.

1. As a result there is a strong SNS stimulation →

    (a) Stronger contraction of the heart
    (b) Increased venous return from blood vessel contraction → leads to a greater RA pressure.

2. Retention of fluid by the kidneys.

    (a) Decreased GFR → RAAS system → aldosterone secretion → Na^+ and water retention.

Move up the Frank-starling curve. However get to the stage where atria are over stretched and the muscle fibers cannot contract efficiently (Fig. 3.12).
Characterised by decreased EF and therefore lower SV, changes in myosin to have slower contraction resulting in a higher end systolic and end diastolic volume.
Systolic failure – characterized by the loss of normal contraction.
Diastolic failure – characterized by loss of normal relaxation.

3 Cardiovascular Physiology

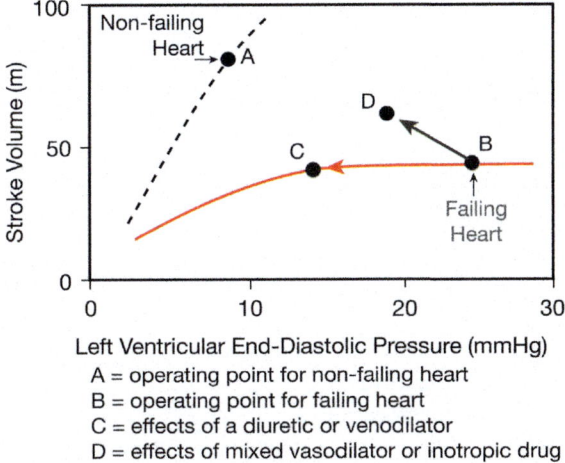

A = operating point for non-failing heart
B = operating point for failing heart
C = effects of a diuretic or venodilator
D = effects of mixed vasodilator or inotropic drug

Fig. 3.12 Effect of heart failure on stroke volume

Shock
Generalised cellular hypoxia from inadequate perfusion, ranging from reversible to irreversible stages
Categories of shock:

- Hypovolemic – from bleeding, burns, GI losses
- Distributive – generalised vasodilation which may be from anaphylaxis or sepsis or neurogenic (↓ sympathetic nerves)
- Cardiogenic – 1′ pump failure from MI, myocarditis, or metabolic, electrolyte disturbances
- Obstructive – from ↓ CO 2′ to external interference (tamponade, tensions pneumothorax, PE)

Compensatory reaction to haemorrhagic shock

- If blood loss → ↓ venous return → ↓ EDV → ↓ SV → ↓ CO → ↓ MABP

  – Baroreceptors will ↓ activity, chemoreceptors will ↑ activity

- Immediate compensation

  – ↑ Sympathetic output → ↑ HR, generalised vasoconstriction

    ↑ TPR → normalises BP but hypoperfusion

      ↓ GI function, oliguria, coldness, ↑ sympathetic activity

  – ↑ Secretion of A, NA (→ as above, plus restlessness)
  – ↑ Secretion of ADH/vasopressin
  – ↑ Secretion of renin → ↑ ATII → ↑ aldosterone → ↑ in BV

- Intermediate
  - ↓ Ultrafiltration (1/2 L of interstitial fluid may be absorbed = internal transfusion)
    - This is increased by the presence of glucose
- Longer term
  - ↑ intake of fluid (through thirst)
  - Release of albumin
  - ↑ EPO → ↑ RBC

  Refractory Shock may result

- Initial precapillary sphincter contraction → hypoxic → relax
- Cell injury → release of free radicals
- Gut injury → bacterial translocation
- ↓ BF to the brain may suppress CVS control mechanisms
- ↓ Myocardial function → decompensation (esp. with ↑ HR and ↑ contractility, lactic acidosis)
- May lead to multiple organ dysfunction syndrome (MODS) → irreversible stage → ↓ CO → hypotension → worsening metabolic state
  - Gross hypoperfusion and extensive necrosis

3.4 Blood Pressure

Questions

1. What are the determinants of blood pressure?
   CO and TPR
2. Where are the main baroreceptors located and what nerve innervates the carotid sinus?
   Carotid sinus near the carotid bifurcation. ('Hering nerve' which is a branch of glossopharyngeal CNIX)
   Aortic arch (vagus CNX).
3. Where is the vasomotor center located?
   The medulla.
4. Where is renin produced?
   In the epitheliod, granular and juxtaglomerular cells of the kidney. It is an enzyme that converts angiotensinogen to angiotensin I.
5. What are the actions of angiotensin II?

   (a) ↑ Na absorption in the proximal tubule
   (b) ↑ secretion of aldosterone (zona glomerulosa of adrenal cortex)
      - Aldosterone → ↑ Na reabsorption from 2nd part of the distal tubule and collecting duct

3 Cardiovascular Physiology   73

    (c) ↓ medullary BF → ↑ Na reabsorption
    (d) ↑ sensitivity of JG feedback
    (e) Potent vasoconstrictor and facilitates NA release, and ↓ vagal tone
    (f) Acts on circumventricular organs in the brain → ↑ BP, ↑ thirst, ↑ ADH and ACTH

6. What is the role of atrial natriuretic peptide (ANP)?
   This is a peptide hormone released by the cardiac muscle cells in response to increased extracellular fluid (ECF). It works by causing natriuresis.

7. What is the oxygen consumption of skeletal muscle at rest?
   It is 250 mL/min and this can increase to 1600 mL/min in hard work.

Blood pressure

Blood pressure is measured with a sphygmomanometer.
As blood is pumped out of the left ventricle into the aorta and distributing arteries, pressure is generated. As the ventricle relaxes, the pressure in the aorta decreases. This is measured as the systolic and diastolic BP.
Blood pressure is determined by CO and TPR. These can be manipulated to maintain or alter blood pressure. The MABP is normally controlled within a narrow range to ensure adequate blood flow through the organs.
The short-term controls involve reflexes integrated in the brain, with long-term control being by factors affecting blood volume.

Medullary Controls

- Peripheral receptors → nucleus of tractus solitarius
  - Includes: Arterial baroreceptors, cardiopulmonary, arterial chemoreceptors, pulmonary stretch and skeletal muscle receptors
  - May relay to vagal motor neurons (nucleus ambiguous and dorsal motor nucleus) or the C1 group for sympathetic excitement

Higher Centres

- Brainstem: Feedback center from baro- and chemoreceptors.
  - Many sites in the reticular substance and hypothalamus can stimulate or inhibit the CVS regulatory neurons in the vasomotor center in the medulla
- Cerebellum helps to regulate the cardiovascular system (CVS) during exercise
- Cerebral cortex also plays a role, most likely through hypothalamus or limbic system

Autonomic nervous system control

- Vasomotor centre in the medulla-
  - Parasympathetic nervous system (PSNS) via the vagus to the heart
  - Sympathetic nervous system (SNS) to the spinal cord to all arteries, arterioles and veins the body. The SNS exerts tonic control over blood vessels.
    - Act via the SNS nerves, which release noradrenaline, which act on $\alpha 1$ receptors of vascular smooth muscle to cause vasoconstriction.

- Nerves that act on the adrenal medulla stimulate release of adrenaline (80%) and noradrenaline (20%)
- Dopamine acts on α, β1, β2 as well as dopaminergic receptors.

Baroreceptor reflex

- Sensors: Baroreceptors: (1) Carotid sinus (located at bifurcation of internal and external carotid) and the (2) Aortic arch baroreceptors.
- Afferent nerves: Carotid sinus- 'Hering nerve' a branch of CNIX, glossopharyngeal
- Aortic arch- CNX, vagus
- These nerves synapse on the nucleus tractus solitarius (NTS)
- Carotid sinus responds to pressure between 60 and 180 mmHg
- If ↑ BP, ↑ stretch of baroreceptors, ↑ baroreceptor firing, travels along NTS to vasomotor center in medulla, ↓ SNS firing and ↑ PSNS firing → ↓ BP

Arterial Chemoreceptors (kick in for ↓ BP)

- Located in the carotid and aortic bodies (highest blood flow per tissue weight of any organ)
- Normally involved with ventilation, but can affect the CVS.
- Afferent nerves join 'Hering nerve' before entering glossopharyngeal nerve
- Hypoxia, hypercapnia or acidosis → ↑ firing → ↓ heart rate and ↑ peripheral vasoconstriction
- In cases of severe ↓ MABP (70) → ↓ flow through chemoR → ↑ SNS → Vasoconstrictor and ↑ HR

Long term control of blood flow and BP
Blood flow:

- The size and number of blood vessels may change appropriately
- Most important stimulus is probably a chronic demand for O_2 → stimulates angiogenic factors

Blood pressure:
This is achieved through altering (1) total blood volume and (2) RBC volume

1. This is achieved through alterations in the kidney, mainly around Na^+ and water handling.

- Initial control of renal handling of sodium is through autoregulation of GFR and tubuloglomerular feedback (*see* Chap. 5)
- Secondary control is through the Renin-Angiotensin-Aldosterone system (RAAS)
    - Renin is an enzyme synthesised by epithelioid, granular and juxtaglomerular cells in the media of the renal glomerular afferent arterioles
    - Renin converts angiotensinogen to Angiotensin I
    - Angiotensin I is converted to Angiotensin II in the lungs by ACE (angiotensin converting enzyme)

- Actions of Angiotensin II
    - Sustained ↓ in BV or ↓ in BP → ↑ AT II production → ↑ in Na^+ retention and ↑ TPR → ↑ ECF, ↑ BP
        - AT II ↑ Na absorption in the proximal tubule
        - AT II ↑ secretion of aldosterone (zona glomerulosa of adrenal cortex)
            o Aldosterone → ↑ Na reabsorption from 2nd part of the distal tubule & collecting duct
        - AT II ↓ medullary BF → ↑ Na reabsorption
        - AT II ↑ sensitivity of JG feedback
        - AT II is a potent vasoconstrictor and facilitates NA release, and ↓ vagal tone
        - AT II acts on circumventricular organs in the brain → ↑ BP, ↑ thirst, ↑ ADH and ACTH
- Control of release
    - Occurs with ↓ in volume, ↓ BP, or ↑ sympathetic output
        - Includes Na^+ depletion, diuretics, hypotension, haemorrhage, upright posture, dehydration, artery constriction, heart failure, cirrhosis
        - Sensed by
            - Renal baroreceptors
            - Macula densa measuring Na^+ and Cl^-
        - Secretion
            - Increased by PGE2 and PGI2
            - Inhibited by ADH, ANP
        - ANP

- 28 a.a. secreted by cardiac muscle cells
- Secretion
    - Increased by ↑ in ECF
    - Decreased by a person standing from being supine
- Actions (opposite to those of RAA system)
    - ↑ renal excretion of Na^+ (natriuretic)
- Control of red cell volume - Erythropoietin
- 165 a.a. glycoprotein secreted by interstitial cells
- 85% from kidneys, 15% from liver
- Action
    - ↓ in O_2 tension → ↑ EPO activity → ↑ number of stem cell to be erythroid
- About ½ of the blood volume is occupied by RBC, therefore plays an important regulatory role in BV

Exercise:
Oxygen consumption and cardiac function

- O_2 consumption at rest is about 250 mL/min, light work 400–800 mL/min, hard work 1600 mL/min.
- Cardiac output rises almost directly with O_2 consumption (from 5 to 20 L/min)
- There is ↑ O_2 uptake from the lungs through ↑ flow and ↑ arteriovenous Δ
- An ↑ in CO is dependent on HR and SV
    - ↑ in HR is initially from ↓ vagal inhibition and then later by ↑ sympathetic discharge
    - ↑ SV is from ↑ filling pressure → ↑ EDV, and ↑ contractility → ↑ EF

Changes in tissue blood flow in exercise

- ↑ Coronary BF
- ↓ and then ~ ↑ through skin
- Vasoconstriction in the splanchnic circulation, kidney and non active muscle
- Vasodilation of skeletal muscle

Training improves transport and utilisation of oxygen in several ways

- Skeletal muscle Δ
    - ↑ extraction, ↓ lactate
    - Growth of new capillaries
    - ↑ in the number of mitochondria
    - ↑ in the quantity of enzymes
    - ↑ concentration of myoglobin
- Heart
    - Ventricular myocardium thickens, ↑ vascularity and cavities enlarge
    - Ventricular EDV may ↑ → ↑ SV → ↓ HR (from vagal inhibition)
    - Leads to up to 7× ↑ in CO

3.5 Control Through Different Circulations

Questions

1. What is the other name for endothelial-derived-relaxing-factor and what is its role?
   It is also known as nitric oxide. It is synthesized from the amino acid L-arginine and it a powerful vasodilator.

2. What is the function of thromboxane A2?
   It acts as a vasoconstrictor as well as promoting platelet aggregation.

3 Cardiovascular Physiology

3. What is the effect of ↑ CO_2 on cerebral circulation?
   The cerebral circulation is very sensitive to carbon dioxide. ↑ CO_2 causes vasodilation and increased cerebral blood flow.

4. Explain the Monro-Kellie doctrine.
   Monro-Kellie doctrine describes the pressure-volume relationship between ICP, volume of CSF, blood, brain tissue, and the cerebral perfusion pressure (CPP). As the skull is fixed, the sum of volumes of brain, CSF, and intracranial blood is constant. An increase in one should cause a decrease in one or both of the remaining two.

5. What is the blood flow of the cerebral circulation per minute?
   750 mL/min.

6. What is the main function of the blood flow to the skin?
   As the skin has a low metabolic demand, its main function is for temperature regulation.

7. In the fetal circulation, where does blood entering the heart from the IVC get preferentially directed?
   This is the blood with the highest oxygen content, hence it is preferentially shunted through the foramen ovale to the left side of the heart, where it is directed to the fetal brain and arms.

8. What causes closure of the foramen ovale at birth?
   This is due to the loss of resistance in the pulmonary circulation when the first breath is taken, as well as a rise in the left atrial pressure due to the rise in systemic pressure when the umbilical cord is cut.

Control through different circulations (Fig. 3.13)
Summary: Local control is achieved in the short term by changes in basal tone, with long term control being made possible by alterations in the size and number of blood vessels
Factors controlling blood flow:
Tissue metabolism

- ↑ metabolism → local changes → SM relaxation → ↑ BF
   - hypoxia and ADP → stimulate EDRF/NO derived from L-arginine.
   - adenosine → ↓ influx of Ca^{2+} ions into SM
   - Acidosis → inactivates calcium channels

- If BF is restored following a period of ischaemia → there is an ↑ in BF (reactive hyperaemia)
   - May be due to accumulation of vasodilator metabolites (e.g. prostaglandins)

Physical Factors

- Temperature
   - ↑ in temperature → vasodilation
   - ↓ in temperature → vasoconstriction
   - At temperatures below 10°C there may be paradoxical vasodilation

Humoral factors
Vasodilation

- Histamine released from basophils and mast cells → powerful arteriolar dilator
- Prostacyclin (arachidonic acid (AA) derivative from COX in endothelium) → vasodilator, stimulates renin release and inhibits platelet aggregation
- Prostaglandins (AA derivatives)
    - E series → vasodilators (contribute to the inflammatory response)
- Kinins (high molecular weight kininogen derivative from proteases) → powerful vasodilators and increases vessel permeability
    - But cause contraction of visceral SM
    - Also chemotactic for leukocytes
- EDRF (NO) secreted by endothelial cells → vasodilation
    - Produced from L-arginine
    - Is a major player systemically
- Increase in K^+, H^+, CO_2 and Mg^{2+} causes vasodilation.

Vasoconstriction

- ATII → powerful vasoconstrictor, esp of arterioles
- ADH → very potent vasoconstrictor but only minute amounts are secreted
- Serotonin (released from platelets) → potentiates the affect of NA → promotes vasoconstriction
- TXA2 (AA derivative from COX in platelets) → vasoconstriction and promotes aggregation
- Leukotrienes (AA derivatives produced by white cells) → vasoconstriction, margination, diapedesis and ↑ permeability of blood vessels
- Prostaglandins (AA derivatives)
    - F series → vasoconstrictors
- Endothelins (ET-1) → powerful vasoconstrictor
- ↑ Ca causes vasoconstriction

Flow through different circulation (Fig. 3.13)

Cerebral circulation

- Arteries include internal carotid artery → anterior cerebral and middle cerebral (each supplies the ant 2/3rd of the cerebral hemisphere) and vertebral → basilar → posterior cerebral (supplies the posterior 1/3rd cerebral hemisphere, brain stem and cerebellum). Together these form the Circle of Willis.
- Venous blood drains mainly to the internal jugular vein + ophthalmic, pterygoid, emissary and paravertebral veins

Region	Mass (kg)	Blood Flow		Arteriovenous Oxygen Difference mL/L	Oxygen Consumption		Resistance (R units)*		Percentage of Total	
		mL/min	mL/100 g/min		mL/min	mL/100 g/min	Absolute	per kg	Cardiac Output	Oxygen Consumption
Liver	2.6	1500	57.7	34	51	2.0	3.6	9.4	27.8	20.4
Kidneys	0.3	1260	420.0	14	18	6.0	4.3	1.3	23.3	7.2
Brain	1.4	750	54.0	62	46	3.3	7.2	10.1	13.9	18.4
Skin	3.6	462	12.8	25	12	0.3	11.7	42.1	8.6	4.8
Skeletal muscle	31.0	840	2.7	60	50	0.2	6.4	198.4	15.6	20.0
Heart muscle	0.3	250	84.0	114	29	9.7	21.4	6.4	4.7	11.6
Rest of body	23.8	330	1.4	129	44	0.2	16.1	383.2	6.2	17.6
Whole body	63.0	5400	8.6	46	250	0.4	1.0	63.0	100.0	100.0

*R units are pressure (mmHg) divided by blood flow (mL/s)
Reproduced with permission from Bard P (editor): *Medical Physiology*, 11th ed. Mosby, 1961

Fig. 3.13 Circulations throughout the body

- Blood brain barrier: Capillary endothelium is relatively impermeable to anything other than H_2O, respiratory gases and some lipid soluble substances
    - This plays a protective role (chemical Δ and infections)
    - Achieved via tight junctions and few cytoplasmic vesicles
- Cerebral blood flow is approx 50–55 mL/100 g/min = 15% CO
    - BF is greater to grey matter than white matter, and local flow ↑ with ↑ metabolic activity
- Total BF depends on BP, venous pressure, ICP, blood viscosity and arteriolar tone
    - Cerebral arteries show considerable autoregulation
    - Very sensitive to $\Delta CO_2 \rightarrow \uparrow CO_2 \rightarrow$ vasodilation and $\downarrow O_2 \rightarrow$ vasodilation
- Vessels are innervated with sympathetic (NA) and cholinergic fibres (ACh, VIP)
- Monro-Kellie doctrine describes the pressure-volume relationship between ICP, volume of CSF, blood, brain tissue, and the cerebral perfusion pressure (CPP). As the skull is fixed, the sum of volumes of brain, CSF, and intracranial blood is constant. An increase in one should cause a decrease in one or both of the remaining two.

Coronary circulation

- Arteries include left coronary artery →
    - Anterior descending branch → AV wall and interventricular septum
    - Circumflex → lateral and posterior parts of the LV
- And right coronary artery → AV groove to atria and right ventricle
    - Posterior descending artery → posterior and inferior parts of the ventricles
- Large arteries lying on the surface give rise to smaller arteries which penetrate the myocardium
    - Myocardium has more capillaries than skeletal muscle
    - Most venous blood → coronary sinus → RA
- Inner 1/10 mm of endocardial surface obtains nutrition from the cardiac chambers.
- Coronary BF at rest is between 70 and 80 mL/100 g/min = 4–5% resting CO
    - In strenuous exercise this may increase by 6–8×, although flow only ↑ by 4× (the remainder due to ↑ efficiency)
- There is a reduction in flow in systole, 80% occurs in diastole (Fig. 3.14).
- The reduction is more pronounced on the left side due to the higher pressures generated

Fig. 3.14 Blood flow in the coronary arteries

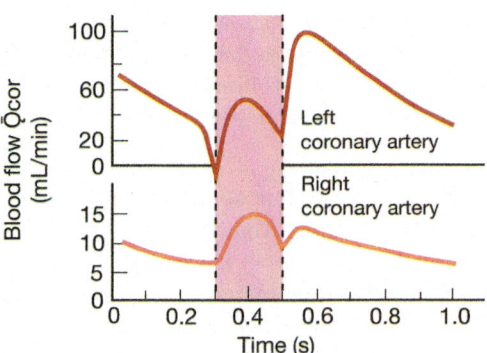

- Control of flow
  - ↑ CO_2, ↑ H^+, ↑ K^+, ↑ lactate, ↑ PG, ↑ adenosine → vasodilation
  - Arterioles are supplied by sympathetic and parasympathetic

Skeletal muscle circulation

- Muscle
  - Red, 15%, tonically active, maintenance of posture
  - White, 85%, phasic activity for movement, have a low resting BF, which can ↑ 20× → 80–90% of CO

- Control of Flow
  - Skeletal muscles arterioles are under tonic sympathetic discharge

    Decrease in the tonic discharge can occur just before exercise
    Once exercise has started though, most control is from local metabolic vasodilation from hypoxia.

  - Dilation ↓ the distance of diffusion and ↑ the area
  - ↑ Hydrostatic pressure → ↑ ultrafiltration → loss of up to 15–20% of plasma volume
  - Flow is ↓ by ↑ pressure generated from the surrounding muscle (0 flow if pressure >70%) → phasic flow

Skin circulation

- Metabolic requirements are small, with the main function being heat regulation (flow varies from 1 to 200 mL/100 g/min)
- Vessels are structured with direct connections between arterioles and venules (coiled and under tonic contraction)
  - ↑ temp → ↓ firing → dilation → ↑ heat loss
- At temperatures below 10°C → paradoxical cold vasodilation may occur (? Temporary cessation of noradrenaline transmission)

- Widespread activation of the sympathetic system in hypovolemic shock → cutaneous vasoconstriction → pale, cold, clammy skin
- White reaction (following light touch) → contraction of precapillary sphincters
- If blood flow is temporarily occluded and then restored → reactive hyperaemia

Fetal circulation
Lungs are non functional, use placenta for gas exchange and removal of excreta.
Blood returning from placenta → umbilical vein → ductus venous → IVC → RA → foramen ovale → LA → LV.
Blood returning in the SVC get preferentially directed to the RV → lungs.
This allows the well oxygenated blood from the placenta to get preferentially directed to the brain.
Changes at birth:
Loss of placental blood flow increases systemic vascular resistance + pulmonary vascular resistance is greatly decreased when first breath is taken.
Resultant change is low pressure in right atrium and high pressure in left atrium, shuts the foramen ovale.
The ductus arteriosus closes due to reversal in blood flow from aorta to pulmonary system. This increases the oxygenation of blood flowing through ductus arteriosus (PaO_2 from 15 mHg to 100 mmHg) and loss of prostaglandin E2.
Ductus Venosus – blood flow through the umbilical vein ceases and the ductus venosus contracts, diverting blood through the liver.

3.6 Flow, Arteries, Veins and Lymph

Questions

1. Use Poiseuille's law to describe the factors determining the resistance to flow.
   Resistance = $8\eta l/\Pi r^4$
   This means that resistance is proportional to the viscosity and the length, and inversely proportional to the radius ^4. As can be seen from the equation, the most important factor determining the resistance to flow is the radius of the vessel.

2. What offers higher resistance to flow – laminar or turbulent flow?
   Turbulent.

3. Over which Reynolds number is flow more likely to be turbulent.
   2000.

   $$Re = velocity \times diameter \times density / viscosity$$

4. What is a Newtonian fluid? Is blood a Newtonian fluid?
   This is when a fluid has a viscosity that is independent of the shear rate. No, blood is not an example of a Newtonian fluid.

3 Cardiovascular Physiology   83

5. Are veins or arteries more distensible?
   Veins. On average 8× more distensible. This is why they are called 'capacitance' vessels and can hold 60% of the blood volume.

6. Describe the law of Laplace and how it relates to the left ventricle.
   This law states that wall tension is proportional to the pressure times radius and inversely proportional to wall thickness. This is why a thin, dilated left ventricle has to generate more wall tension than a hypertrophied LV.

7. Is there pulsatile flow in the capillaries?
   No, due to the compliance of the arterial tree the pressure of pulsations is usually decreased by the time that the blood reaches the capillary so that flow is not pulsatile at all.

8. What would happen to venous return if peripheral venous pressure = CVP?
   See Fig. 3.17.
   There would be no venous return. This is because venous return relies on an incremental fall in pressure to allow blood to return to the heart.

9. In which part of the body are there specific blood reservoirs?
   (1) Spleen (2) Liver (3) Large abdominal veins (4) Venous plexus beneath the skin

10. What is the total lymph production per day?
    2–3 L. This is of high importance as proteins can not be absorbed from the tissues in any other way.

11. Name some conditions that interfere with lymph flow.
    Anything that effects Starlings equilibrium e.g. high venous pressure, low oncotic pressure in capillaries, interstitial fluid pressure, increased permeability and exercise which acts as a pump to lymphatic flow.

Volumes, Areas, Flows and Pressures

- At rest there is 4× more blood in the systemic veins (64%) than the systemic arteries (16%)
  - 8% in the heart, 8% in the lungs, 5% in the capillaries
- Average aorta cross section is 4–5 cm^2, arterioles 400 cm^2, capillaries 4500 cm^2
- Arterioles are the main site of resistance (about 45%)
- Resistance in the pulmonary circulation of about 10% of the systemic circulation

Blood Flow
Depends on *pressure difference* between the two ends and the *vascular resistance*
Arterial distensibility allows intermittent cardiac output to translate to a more continuous flow in capillaries

Aortic pressure

- Shows an initial sharp rise to reach to systolic pressure
- Decreasing ventricular output then equals peripheral run off
- Dicrotic notch occurs from closure of the aortic valve
- As blood continues to run off the pressure continues to decrease

- Pulse pressure = systolic pressure − diastolic pressure
- MABP = diastolic + 1/3 (systolic pressure − diastolic pressure)
- Arterial pressure wave travels much faster than the actual blood
    - 3–5 ms^{-1} in the aorta, 7–10 ms^{-1} large arteries, 15–35 ms^{-1} in small arteries
    - Slower in the elastic aorta and faster in the less distensible smaller arteries
    - Pressure transmission ↑ with age with the loss of elastic tissue
- The change in pulse pressure with inspiration and expiration is not normally detectable
    - If so, pulses paradoxus – seen in asthma and cardiac tamponade
- Abnormally steep or large pulse pressures may be seen in patients AV insufficiency
- ↑ in SBP in age is explained by the ↓ in distensibility
- MABP is determined by CO × TPR

Systemic BP = 120/80 mmHg = average 100 mmHg
Pulmonary BP = 25/8 = average 16 mmHg
However total blood flow through them per minute is equal.

Resistance
The total pulmonary vascular resistance is much less than the systemic circulation. Poiseuille's Equation (see Chap. 4 for further explanation)

- Factors contributing to resistance include viscosity, length of tube, radius
- Resistance = $8\eta l/\Pi r^4$
- Where n = viscosity, l = length and r = radius.
    - NOTE that this is radius to the ^4,

Laminar and Turbulent Flow

- When flow is laminar, there is a stationary film at the edge with a parabolic increase in flow towards the centre (Fig. 3.15).
- With such flow, the shear stress will be force/area
    - If a fluid has a viscosity independent of shear rate then it is said to be Newtonian
        - Blood is NOT Newtonian, with its viscosity INCREASING at lower flow rates
        - In capillaries this does not apply as the cells all align due to the narrow diameter
        - Viscosity of blood depends on the haematocrit and plasma proteins

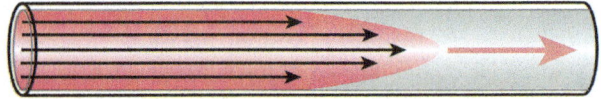

Fig. 3.15 Laminar flow

3 Cardiovascular Physiology

- Flow is more likely to become turbulent when the Reynolds number exceeds 2000

$$Re = velocity \times diameter \times density / viscosity$$

  - For blood the critical velocity is about 40 cm s^{-1}

Law of Laplace

- This states that the wall tension (T) is proportionate to the pressure (P) × radius (r) for thin walled spheres or cylinders.
  - Essentially a larger vessel will have a greater outward distending force than a smaller vessel
  - APPLICATIONS:
    - A capillary can withstand a transmural pressure ¼ of the aorta
    - A dilated heart has to do much more work to overcome the larger tension

Veins

Veins are conduits, but due to their high distensibility they can also store large volumes of blood. Flow is by muscular pumps and valves regulate the direction.

Venous Pressures and Flows

Central Venous Pressure (CVP) can range from −5 to 30 mmHg.

- Can be measured by pulmonary artery flotation catheters, which also measure pulmonary artery wedge pressure (surrogate marker for left sided pressure) and cardiac index.

Effects of Gravity

- Venous pressures are affected by gravity (0.77 mmHg/cm from the heart)
  - Venous blood may be +85 to 90 mmHg at the feet and sub atmospheric in the brain (Fig. 3.16).
  - 15–20% of the blood volume may pool in the legs of someone standing still → syncope when standing for long periods of time.

Factors promoting venous return

- Skeletal muscle contraction → ↑ venous return (reduces effective venous pressure to about 25–30 mmHg)
- During inspiration the intrathoracic pressure decreases → promotes venous return
- Cardiac action (RA pressure ↓ during ventricular systole) → ↑ venous return

Venous return curves

- VR, CVP and CO is closely interrelated (Fig. 3.17).
  - At resting state

    If CVP = peripheral venous pressure (7 mmHg) venous return will be 0
    A decrease in CVP will ↑ venous return

  - ↓ in resistance steepens the curve, ↑ in resistance flattens the curve

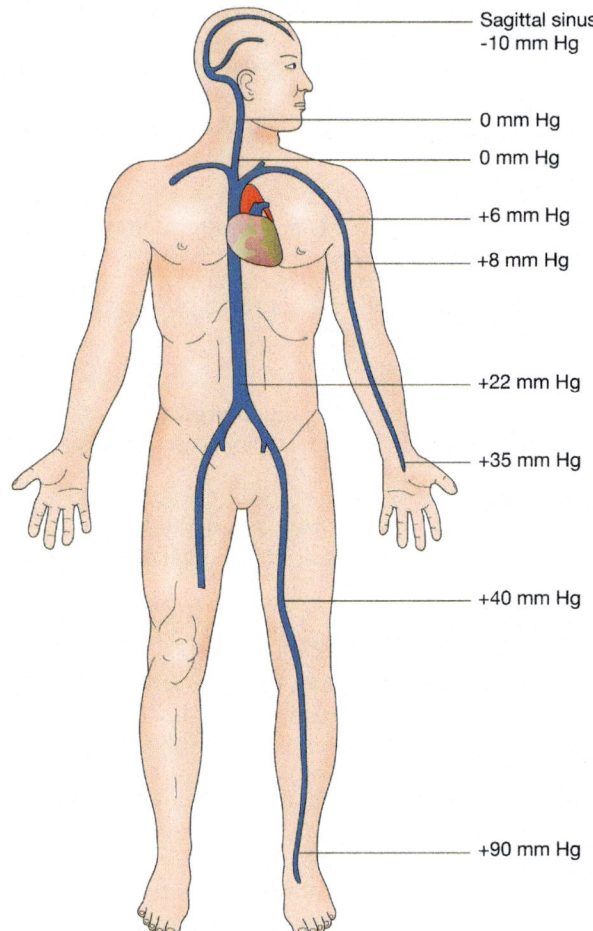

Fig. 3.16 Venous return vs cardiac output

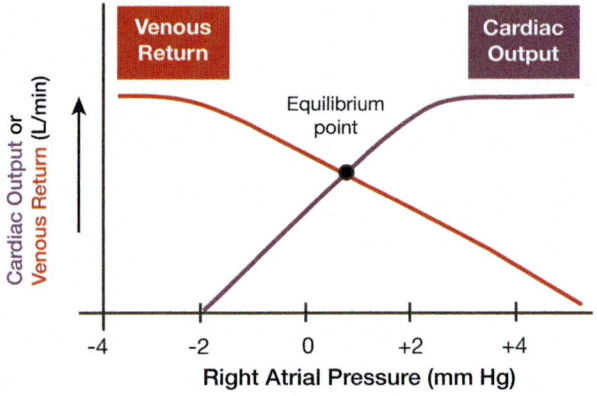

Fig. 3.17 Venous pressure

3 Cardiovascular Physiology

Capillaries

- About ten billion capillaries provide a vast area for diffusion
- Few cells will be further than 20–30 μm from a capillary

Structure

- Nutrient artery → six to eight branches → arteriole (20–30 μm diameter) → metarterioles → SM cuff (precapillary sphincter) → capillaries → venules (richly innervated)

Exchange between blood and interstitial fluid

- Substances move across capillary walls by diffusion (down concentration gradients)
- Lipid soluble substances can pass directly through plasma membranes
- Water and lipo-phobic substances pass through pores, usually 6–7 nm.
  - The size of these pores varies greatly between tissues, but generally does not let proteins through

Interstitial Fluid

- Gel of glycosaminoglycans (GAG's) and proteoglycans
- Pressure inside the interstitial fluid is composed of hydrostatic and osmotic factors

Starling Equilibrium

- Loss of fluid by osmosis is almost completely balanced by return (Fig. 3.18)
- Early on fluid moves out by hydrostatic pressures, and then later returns by colloid osmotic pressure
  - Intravascular colloid osmotic pressure is about 28 mmHg (19 from proteins and 9 from associated inorganic ions)

  Tissue osmotic pressure is about 3 → hence a difference of about 25 mmHg

  - Hydrostatic pressure varies from about 30–32 → 15–17

  Therefore net outward force initially and then a net inward force

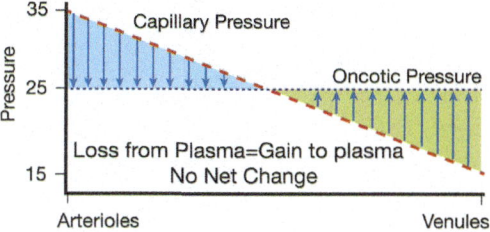

Fig. 3.18 Fluid shift

- About 16 mL/min flows out and 14 mL/min flow in → leaving a net of 2 mL/min as lymph

  These flows are very small compared with blood flows of about 5000 mL/min

- This allows for some control → if BP ↓ then ↓ hydrostatic pressures and ↓ ultrafiltration

- This is also dependent on the capillary filtration coefficient.

Lymphatics
- Supplements the venous system
- Lymphatic capillaries have one-way valves
- Surrounding movement ↑ flow.
- Larger lymphatics have smooth muscle in the walls
- Normally flow is about 2 mL/min; this ↑ dramatically with exercise

Chapter 4
Respiratory Physiology

S. Ali Mirjalili, Lucy Hinton, and Kevin Ellyett

4.1 Structure and Function

Short notes

- Lungs primary function is gas exchange, but also performs other roles i.e. metabolism, filter, blood reservoir
- Surface area is significantly increased due to multiple small units
- Lung volume is increased by the descent of the diaphragm and contraction of the intercostal muscles, scalenes and sternocleidomastoid
- Pulmonary circulation has amazingly low resistance
- Surfactant significantly increases the stability of the alveoli and reduces the work of breathing
- Alveoli have no cilia, hence particles are engulfed by macrophages or moved to ciliated airways utilising the effect of surfactant

Details

- Blood gas barrier is exceedingly thin and has a surface area of 50–100 m^2
- About 300 million alveoli in the human lung

- Terminal bronchioles are the smallest airways without alveoli, further distal is the acinus
- Conducting airways constitute anatomic dead air space (~150 mL)
- Diameter of the capillary segment is about 10 mm → just large enough for an RBC
- Each RBC traverses the capillary bed in 0.75 s

4.2 Ventilation

Questions

1. What are the normal spirometry values expected for a 70 kg adult male?

    (a) Inspiratory reserve volume (IRV)
    (b) Expiratory reserve volume (ERV)
    (c) Tidal volume (TV)

    IRV 3500 mL
    ERV 1000 mL
    TV 500 mL

2. What is the functional residual capacity (FRC) of the lung?
    FRC is the volume left in the lung at the end of quiet expiration. It is equal to the expiratory reserve volume plus the residual volume. It represents the volume at which the want of the chest wall to spring out matches the want of the lung to recoil inwards.

3. What is anatomical dead space? How can it be measured?
    Volume of gas in the conducting airways that does not take part in gas exchange; ~150 mL. Measured using Fowler's method.

4. What is physiological dead space? How can it be measured?
    This is the volume of lung that is not cleared of CO_2. Made up of the anatomical dead space plus the poorly perfused alveoli where there is ventilation without gas exchange (alveolar dead space). Measured using Bohr's method.
    In health there is little difference between the anatomical dead space and the physiological dead space. However, in disease states the physiological dead space may be considerably larger than anatomical dead space.

5. Functional residual capacity (FRC) can be altered by different disease states; name three conditions where FRC is increased?
    FRC is the lung volume at the end of quiet expiration (end of tidal volume). This can be increased by emphysema, positive pressure ventilation as well as going from supine position to standing.

6. A patient's P_{ACO2} rises from 40 mmHg to 80 mmHg. What has happened to their alveolar ventilation?

It has halved. This is because alveolar ventilation and P_{ACO2} are inversely proportional.

7. What three lung volume values can not be measured with spirometry?
Residual volume, functional residual capacity and total lung capacity. The residual volume can not be measured with spirometry. This means that both the functional residual capacity and the total lung capacity can not be measured with spirometry as these capacities contain the residual volume in their measurement.

Short notes

- A spirometer (Fig. 4.1) is commonly used to measure lung volumes.

Measurement	What it measures	Normal value for 70 kg male
Tidal volume (TV)	Amount of air entering lungs during quiet breathing	~500 mL
Inspiratory reserve volume (IRV)	Maximal amount of additional air that can be inhaled after normal inspiration	~3500 mL
Expiratory reserve volume (ERV)	Maximal amount of air that can be exhaled from the lungs after normal expiration	~1000 mL
Residual volume (RV)	Amount of air left in the lungs after maximal expiration	~1200 mL
Vital capacity (VC)	From maximum inspiration of maximum expiration. The sum of TV, IRV and ERV	~5000 mL
Total lung capacity (TLC)	The sum of TV, IRV, ERV and RV	~6000 mL
Inspiratory capacity (IC)	Amount of air that can be inhaled at the end of quiet expiration. IRV + TV	~4000 mL
Functional residual capacity (FRC)	Amount remaining after normal expiration. It is when the chest wall's want to 'spring out' equal to the lungs want to 'recoil'	~2200 mL

Spirometry can measure inspiratory reserve volume (IRV), tidal volume (TV) and expiratory reserve volume (ERV) (and therefore VC, IC).

Spirometry can not measure residual volume (RV), hence need to use nitrogen wash-out, gas dilutional method or whole body plesmethography to measure RV and hence FRC and TLC.

Ventilation and dead space

Total ventilation = Volume of air inhaled each breath (TV) × breaths per minute

Alveolar ventilation = Volume of gas entering the alveolar. This is less than total ventilation due to anatomical dead space (see below)
- Calculated by amount entering respiratory zone × breaths per minute
- Alveolar ventilation can be increased by increasing tidal volume or frequency (or both)
- CO_2 is a good indicator of alveolar ventilation (not produced in the dead space)

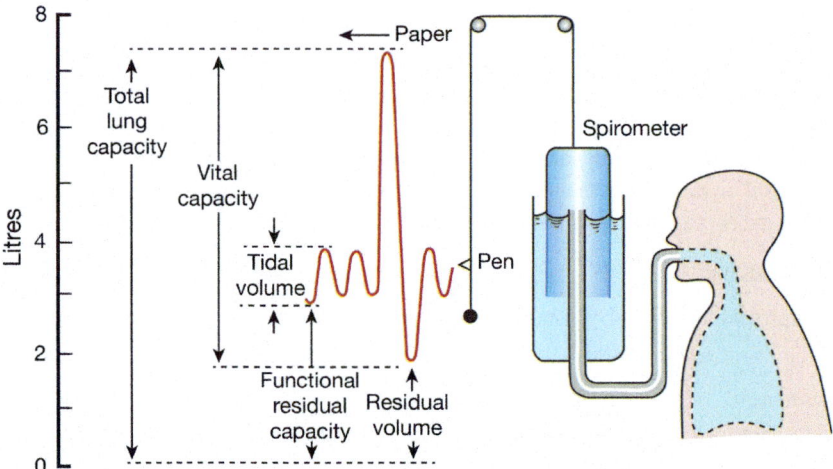

Fig. 4.1 Spirometer with lung measurements

- Arterial and alveolar CO_2 are near identical, so arterial CO_2 reflects alveolar ventilation; if alveolar ventilation is halved, the arterial CO_2 will double

  Anatomical dead space = Volume of air in the conducting airways that does not take part in gas exchange (~150 mL)

- Measured by Fowler's method- Measures the volume of the conducting airways where rapid dilution of inspired gas mixes with remaining gas

  Physiologic dead space = This is air that does not take part in gas exchange as it is in the conducting airways PLUS air in alveoli that are poorly perfused. i.e. measures the volume of the lung that does not eliminate CO_2

- Measured by Bohr's method
- In health anatomical and physiological dead space are roughly equal, however in diseased lungs with $\dot{V}/\dot{Q}$ mismatching physiological dead space can increase

4.3 Diffusion

Questions

1. What is the surface area of the lung? What is the blood-gas barrier thickness?
   50–100 m^2
   0.3 μm

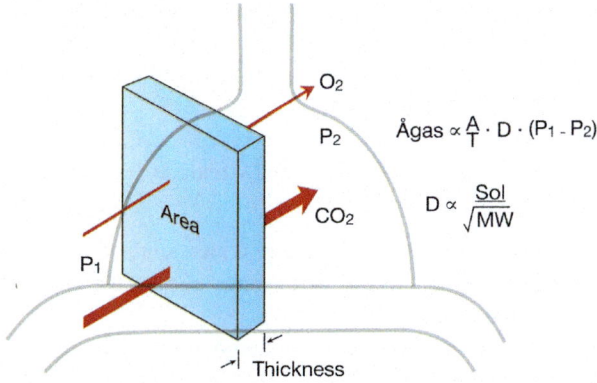

Fig. 4.2 Components of Fick's law of diffusion

Use this to explain why the lung is so well design for oxygenation of blood?
This is because diffusion of a gas follows 'Fick's law of diffusion' where the rate of diffusion is proportional to the area (large) and inversely proportional to the thickness (small) (Fig. 4.2)

2. Why does CO_2 diffuse more quickly than O_2?
This is because CO_2 is 20 times more soluble than O_2, and therefore has a higher diffusion constant. Diffusion constant $\propto$ solubility/square root of molecular weight.

3. A patient is admitted with shortness of breath due to severe pulmonary fibrosis. In pulmonary fibrosis, which component of Fick's law is altered?
The blood-gas thickness is increased in pulmonary fibrosis. As diffusion is inversely proportional to thickness, diffusion is slower (Fig. 4.2).

4. Give an example of a gas that is diffusion limited?
Carbon Monoxide. As CO rapidly binds with haemoglobin, the partial pressure of CO in the blood is close to zero, therefore the rate of transfer of CO from the alveolar space into the blood is determined by the partial pressure of alveolar CO and the diffusion capacity of the lung for CO (which is ~80% to that of O_2 and ~4% to that of CO_2). Therefore the rate of the transfer of CO from the alveoli into the blood, for a given lung, is principally determined by the alveolar partial pressure of CO and hence the transfer is diffusion limited.

5. Give an example of a gas that is perfusion limited?
Nitrous oxide. Nitrous oxide rapidly diffuses and is NOT bound by any proteins, resulting in a quick rise in the partial pressure. Therefore equilibrium between the alveoli and capillary is quickly reached, preventing further diffusion, before blood reaches the end of the capillary.

6. Under normal conditions, how long does it take for equilibrium to be established between partial pressure of oxygen in the alveoli and the capillaries?
   0.25 s. This is a third of the normal transit time of blood in the capillaries.

Short notes

Gas in the alveoli needs to reach the blood stream before it can be distributed to body tissues. This happens by the process of diffusion.

- The rate of diffusion follows 'Fick's Law' which states that diffusion is proportional to tissue surface area and the difference in partial pressure, and inversely proportional to tissue thickness
- It also takes into account the 'diffusion constant' which is proportional to gas solubility, and inversely proportional to the square of the gas molecular weight (MW)
- Fick's law with respect to gas exchange

$$\dot{V}_{gas} = -DA \cdot \frac{\Delta P_{gas}}{T}$$

where $\dot{V}$ = rate of gas transfer, D = diffusion coefficient ($\propto$ solubility/$\sqrt{MW}$). ΔP_{gas} = partial pressure gradient across the membrane, T = thickness and A = area (Fig. 4.3).

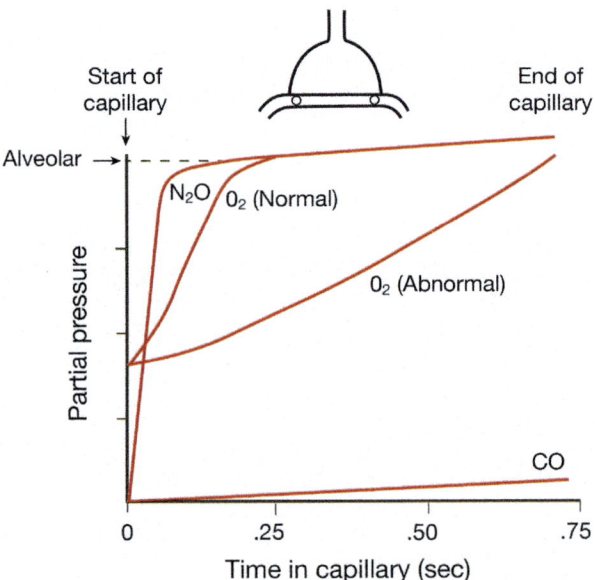

Fig. 4.3 Diffusion (CO) and perfusion (N_2O) limited gases

4 Respiratory Physiology

The rate of diffusion can be diffusion limited, perfusion limited or a combination.

- Diffusion limited reactions are limited by the diffusion properties of the gas e.g. carbon monoxide (CO)
  - Typical of substances which once diffused are rapidly taken up by blood proteins (CO quickly interacts with Hb) therefore its rate of uptake is predominantly determined by its alveolar partial pressure
- Perfusion limited reactions are limited by the amount of blood flow e.g. Nitrous oxide (N_2O)
  - If blood flow increased then more gas would be taken up into the bloodstream
  - Typical of substances which reach saturation rapidly (N_2O is not taken up by Hb hence its partial pressure rises quickly)
- Oxygen behaves somewhere between the two.
- This is because haemoglobin does bind with oxygen, but with less avidity than carbon monoxide. O_2 uptake can be considered to occur as (1) diffusion and (2) reaction with Hb
  - Under normal conditions saturation ($P_{AO2} = P_{c'O2}$) is reached at one third of the way along the capillary (0.25 s) → perfusion limited
  - In severe exercise the time the RBC spends in a capillary can be one third of normal (0.25 s). Under normal conditions, equilibrium will still be reached.
  - Under some disease states diffusion is impaired e.g. increased wall thickness → diffusion limited
  - At low PO_2 (e.g. high altitude), the pressure differential is less therefore arterial saturation may drop
- Diffusion capacity of the lung (D_L) includes area, thickness and diffusion properties of the tissue sheet and gas. CO uptake techniques can be used to measure lung diffusion properties. This is because CO is diffusion limited.

4.4 Blood Flow and Metabolism

Questions

1. What are the two mechanisms whereby pulmonary vascular resistance can be deceased?
   Recruitment and distension of capillaries

2. Describe the changes in lung resistance at different lung volumes?
   At low lung volumes there is high resistance because of loss of radial traction of the extra-alveolar vessels.
   At high lung volumes there is an increase in resistance, as the alveolar pressure exceeds the capillary pressure and therefore squeezes the capillaries shut preventing blood flow.
   At lung volumes close to FRC, the vascular resistance is near its lowest with neither of the aforementioned mechanisms having significant effect (Fig. 4.4).

3. Why is pulmonary vascular resistance increased when there is hypoxia?
   This is due to hypoxic pulmonary vasoconstriction. This mechanism tries to divert blood from the poorly ventilated areas to areas of the lung with better ventilation. The underlying mechanism is unknown, but it is thought to be involved with nitric oxide (NO).

4. How can cardiac output be calculated?
   This can be calculated from Fick's principle, whereby

$$\dot{Q} = \frac{\dot{V}_{O_2}}{\left(C_{aO_2} - C^-_{cO_2}\right)}$$

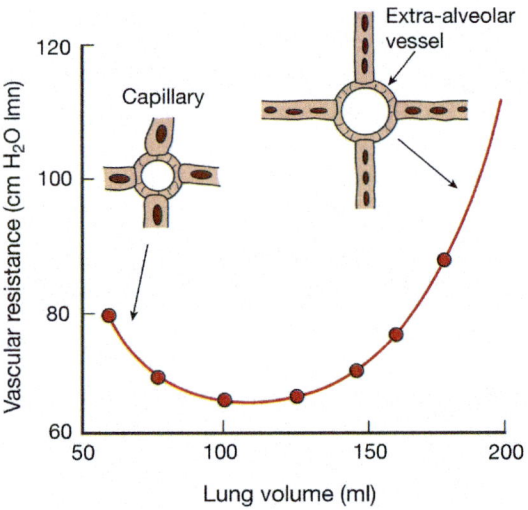

Fig. 4.4 Vascular resistance at different lung volumes

$\dot{Q}$ = cardiac output, $\dot{V}_{O_2}$ = rate of O_2 consumption, C_{aO2} = arterial oxygen content, $\bar{C}_{cO_2}$ = mixed venous oxygen content.

Arterial oxygen content can be measured from an arterial blood sample. Mixed venous oxygen content can be measured from blood from the right atrium sampled via a pulmonary artery catheter. Volume of oxygen consumption is measured by collection and analysis of expired gas.

5. Describe West's zones of the lung Fig. 4.5.

   (a) Zone 1; Upper lung. Where pulmonary arterial pressure falls below alveolar pressure

   - This squashes the capillaries and no blood flow occurs
   - Does not occur normally, but may with haemorrhage or hypotension.
   - This adds to alveolar dead space as ventilated but not perfused.

   (b) Zone 2; Mid lung: Where pulmonary arterial pressure exceeds alveolar pressure, which exceeds venous pressure

   - Blood flow is determined by arterial-alveolar difference

   (c) Zone 3; Lower lung: Where pulmonary artery and venous pressure exceeds alveolar pressure

   - Flow is determined by arterial-venous difference and increased through distension

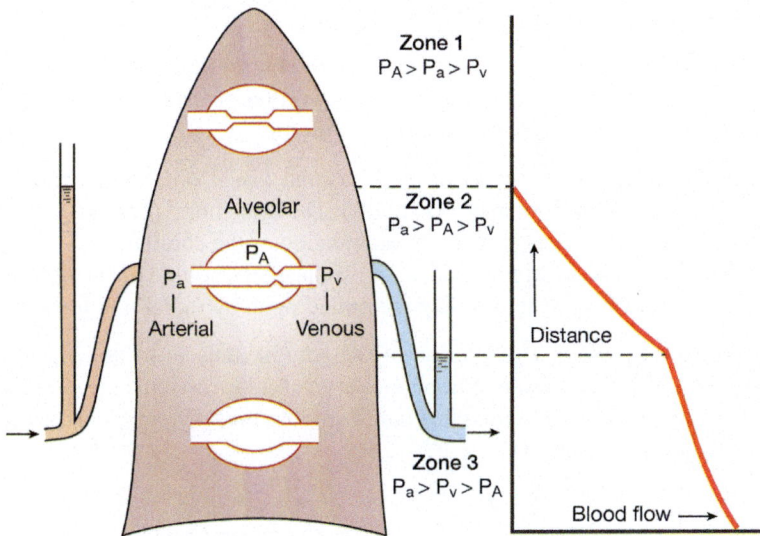

Fig. 4.5 West's zones of the lungs

6. Except for gas exchange, what are some other functions of the lung?

    (a) Metabolism
    (b) Blood filter
    (c) Reservoir for blood
    (d) Vocalisation
    (e) Conversion of angiotensin I to angiotensin II

Short notes

- Pulmonary capillaries form a dense network in the alveolar wall
- Pulmonary system is low pressure
- Mean pressure in the pulmonary artery is only about 15 mmHg (SBP 25/DBP 8) *c.f.* 100 mmHg in the systemic circulation
- Wall of the pulmonary artery is very thin and contains little smooth muscle
- Pulmonary resistance has the ability to decrease with increased pressure

    – This can be done through (1) recruitment and (2) distension
    – Recruitment: When pulmonary arterial blood pressure rises; capillaries that are usually shut, open and conduct blood
    – Distension: At higher vascular pressure, capillaries widen

- Lung volume also influences resistance;

    – At higher volumes the extra-alveolar vessels are held open and their resistance decreases
    – However when alveolar size increases at large lung volumes, there is compression of the surrounding capillaries which increases resistance
    – At low lung volumes there is high resistance due to the small calibre of the extra-alveolar vessels (Fig. 4.4)

- The lung vasculature requires much less local control than systemic circulation
- Alveolar capillaries are greatly affected by alveolar pressure, however the extra-alveolar vessels are affected by total lung volume

    – Capillaries are liable to collapse or distend based on surrounding alveolar pressure (see West's zones of the lungs). The transmural pressure is the difference between the pressure inside and outside of the capillaries
    – The extra-alveolar (arteries and veins) are less susceptible to alveolar pressure and at higher lung volumes they are pulled open by radial traction

- Any factor that causes constriction of the smooth muscle in the extra-alveolar blood vessels will cause a rise in pulmonary vascular resistance (e.g. serotonin)
- The converse is true for factors that cause smooth muscle relaxation (e.g. acetylcholine and isoproterenol)

Hypoxia causes increased vascular resistance, due to the reflex to shunt blood away from hypoxic alveoli, (mainly if the partial pressure of oxygen is less than 70 mmHg), thus increasing the resistance in the blood vessels leading to the hypoxic area

- Believed to occur through NO and L-arginine pathways
- Has the effect of directing blood away from hypoxic region of the lung
- At high altitude generalised pulmonary vasoconstriction can occur
- Important physiological process at birth

- A low blood pH causes vasoconstriction
- Vascular resistance is calculated from Δ pressure/blood flow
- Volume of blood flowing through the lungs each minute can be calculated using Fick's principle:

$$\dot{Q} = \frac{\dot{V}_{O_2}}{\left(C_{aO_2} - C^-_{cO_2}\right)}$$

Arterial oxygen content can be measured from an arterial blood sample. Mixed venous content can be measured from blood from the right atrium sampled via a pulmonary artery catheter. Volume of oxygen consumption is measured by collecting and analysing expired gas.

- Considerable perfusion inequality exists within the human lung, with much less at the top than at the bottom (gravity dependent). These are known as West's zone of the lung.
  - Zone 1; Upper lung. Where pulmonary arterial pressure falls below alveolar pressure
    - This squashes the capillaries and no flow occurs
    - Does not occur normally, but may with haemorrhage or hypotension
    - This adds to alveolar dead space as ventilated but not perfused
  - Zone 2; Mid lung: Where pulmonary arterial pressure exceeds alveolar which exceeds venous pressure
    - Blood flow is determined by arterial-alveolar differences
  - Zone 3; Lower lung: Where pulmonary artery and venous pressure exceeds alveolar pressure
    - Flow is determined by arterial-venous difference and increased through distension (Fig. 4.5)
- Water balance in the lung is dependent on hydrostatic pressure and osmotic pressure (Starling Equation). Fluid that reaches the alveolar spaces is actively pumped out by Na$^+$K$^+$ ATPase in the epithelial cells
- The rate of lymph flow increases considerably with increased capillary pressure

- Other functions of the lung are as a blood reservoir, and blood filter (thrombi)
- Also plays an important metabolic role
    - Converts Angiotensin I to Angiotensin II
    - May activate some amino acids substrates
    - Breaks down bradykinin, 5HT, PGE
    - Likely to be involved in coagulation pathways
    - Important synthetic function of surfactant

4.5 Ventilation-Perfusion Relationship

Questions

1. Calculate the P_{AO_2} at sea level?

$$P_{AO_2} = F_{iO_2} \times (PB - P_{H_2O}) - \frac{P_{aCO_2}}{R}$$
$$= 0.21 \times (760 - 47) - \frac{40}{0.8}$$
$$= 100 \text{ mmHg}$$

2. What are the different percentages of nitrogen, oxygen and carbon dioxide in the atmosphere?
Nitrogen = 78%
Oxygen = 21%
Carbon dioxide = 0.04%.

3. Name five causes of hypoxia.
    (a) Decreased F_{iO2}
    (b) Hypoventilation
    (c) Diffusion abnormality
    (d) Shunt
    (e) Ventilation-perfusion ($\dot{V}/\dot{Q}$) mismatch

4. If a patient hypoventilates, what direction will their CO_2 move?
It will increase. Ventilation is inversely proportional to the amount of CO_2 in the blood. If ventilation halves, then the CO_2 will double.

4 Respiratory Physiology

5. Define a shunt.
   This is blood that exits the right ventricle then exits the left ventricle without undergoing gas exchange.

6. Is a shunt always pathological?
   No. This is because in health, there is a small shunt from the bronchial circulation that does not pass through the ventilated lung tissue. Furthermore, the thebesian veins that drain directly into the left side of the heart contribute to the physiological shunt.

7. Which of the five causes of hypoxia can not be corrected by oxygen therapy?
   Shunt.

8. Is the P_{AO_2} higher at the top or bottom of the lung?
   The Top. This is because there is proportionally higher ventilation but poorer perfusion, meaning less oxygen diffuses from the alveoli into the blood stream, resulting in a higher P_{AO_2}.

<u>Short notes</u>

Oxygen transport in tissue- There is a constant decrease in the partial pressure of oxygen, from the atmosphere to the mitochondria, where it is used in cellular respiration (Fig. 4.6).

- P_{O_2} of inspired air is about 150 mmHg (see alveolar gas equation)
- P_{O_2} of alveolar gas (P_{AO_2}) is about 100 mmHg, this is much less with hypoventilation

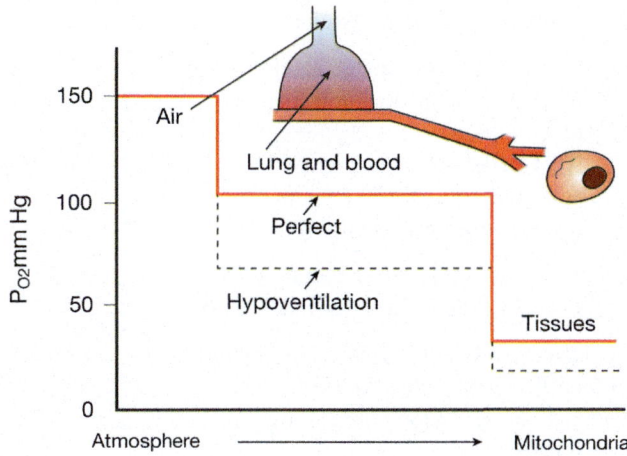

Fig. 4.6 Partial pressure of oxygen

- P_{aO2} = arterial P_{O2}, measured on arterial blood gas
- Normal Alveolar-arterial gradient (A-a gradient) is about 4 mmHg = $P_{AO2} - P_{aO2}$

Causes of hypoxia can fall into groups;

1. Decreased fraction of inspired oxygen
2. Hypoventilation
3. Diffusion abnormality
4. Shunt
5. Ventilation-perfusion mismatch

Hypoventilation results in decreased P_{O2} and increased P_{CO2}

- Results from drugs (morphine, benzodiazepines), sleep disordered breathing, chest wall damage, neuromuscular disorders and high resistance breathing
- If alveolar ventilation is halved, P_{CO2} is doubled
- Values can be calculated by the alveolar gas equation

$$P_{AO_2} = F_{iO_2} \times (P_B - P_{H_2O}) - \frac{P_{aCO_2}}{R}$$

P_B = Barometric Pressure, P_{H2O} = saturated water vapour pressure at 37 °C (47 mmHg).

Diffusion: Alveolar and arterial difference is usually extremely small, but can increase with exercise, disease, or low O_2.

- Shunt: Refers to blood that exits the right ventricle then exits the left ventricle without undergoing gas exchange
  - Caused by (1) bronchial and coronary veins; (2) abnormal vascular connections (e.g. abnormal intrahepatic vascular connections); (3) Right → Left heart defects
  - **NOTE:** Hypoxemia caused by a right to left shunt cannot be abolished by administering 100% oxygen
  - A shunt does not usually result in a raised P_{CO2}

Ventilation/Perfusion mismatch: In all lungs there is ventilation/perfusion mismatch, even in healthy individuals.

- Concentration of O_2 in any lung unit is determined by the ratio of ventilation to blood flow (and other gases)
- Mixed venous blood entering the lungs will have a P_{O2} of 40 mmHg and P_{CO2} of 45 mmHg
- Adequate oxygenation is dependent on addition of O_2 by ventilation and by adequate flow of blood
  - If air flow is decreased → Alveolar O_2 will drop and CO_2 will rise = decreasing $\dot{V}/\dot{Q}$
  - If blood flow is decreased → Alveolar O_2 will rise and CO_2 will drop = increasing $\dot{V}/\dot{Q}$

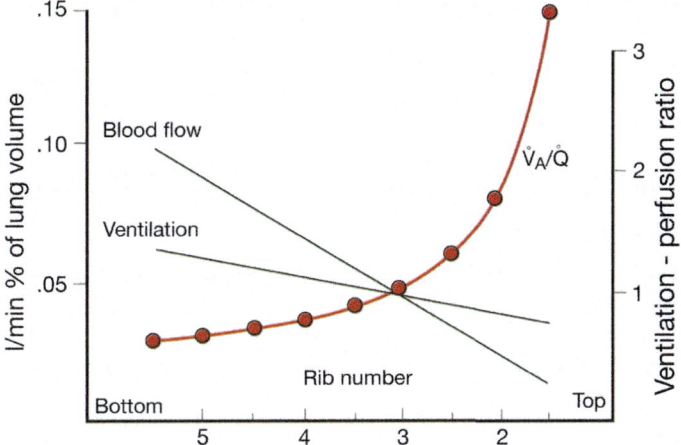

Fig. 4.7 Ventilation-Perfusion relationship in the lungs

- Ventilation decreases slowly from the bottom to the top, blood flow decreases more rapidly (Fig. 4.7)
    - Therefore → ventilation/perfusion ratio is high at the top and low at the bottom
    - P_{O2} of the alveoli decreases significantly from top to bottom (132 → 89 mmHg)
    - P_{CO2} of the alveoli does the opposite
    - Ventilation is still less at the top, but perfusion is even less

4.6 Gas Transport in the Blood

Questions

1. What are the two ways that oxygen can be carried in blood?
   Dissolved and bound to haemoglobin.

2. What globin chains make up adult haemoglobin?
   Two alpha and two beta. Known as haemoglobin A.

3. What form of iron is found in haemoglobin?
   It's ferrous form, Fe^{2+}. If it is Fe^{3+} then it is called methaemoglobinaemia.

4. In venous blood what proportion of carbon dioxide is found 1. Dissolved 2. Bound to Hb as carbaminoHb and 3. Bicarbonate?
   (1) 10%, (2) 30%, (3) 60%

5. In arterial blood what proportion of carbon dioxide is found (1) Dissolved (2) Bound to Hb as carbaminoHb and (3) Bicarbonate?
   (1) 5%, (2) 5%, (3) 90%.

6. Explain the Haldane effect.
   This explains the effect of oxygen on carbon dioxide carriage in the blood. In the peripheries the deoxygenated haemoglobin is able to carry more carbon dioxide. Conversely in the lungs, the loading of oxygen on haemoglobin assists the unloading of carbon dioxide.

7. Does the lung or the kidney have a greater ability to excrete acid?
   The lung. 100 times greater, this is done by altering the ventilation and therefore altering the P_{aCO_2}.

8. Below is the blood gas of a patient presenting acutely unwell to the Emergency Department.

   pH = 7.15.
   P_{CO_2} = 30 mmHg
   P_{O_2} = 100 mmHg
   HCO_3^- = 10 mmol L^{-1}

   What is this consistent with?
   Metabolic acidosis with partial respiratory compensation. This could be consistent with diabetic ketoacidosis.

Short notes

- Oxygen is carried in the blood in two forms: dissolved and combined with Hb
- The amount dissolved obeys Henry's law (amount of gas dissolved in an equilibrium is directly related to the partial pressure of the gas).
- Normal arterial partial pressure of oxygen is around 100 mmHg.
  - For every 1 mmHg of P_{O_2} there is 0.03 mL/L^{-1} of dissolved oxygen, therefore is 3 mL/L^{-1} at normal P_{aO_2} of 100 mmHg. This would mean the average 70 kg man would have ~15 mL of oxygen in their blood. This is not compatible with life.
  - Therefore need Haemoglobin (Hb);

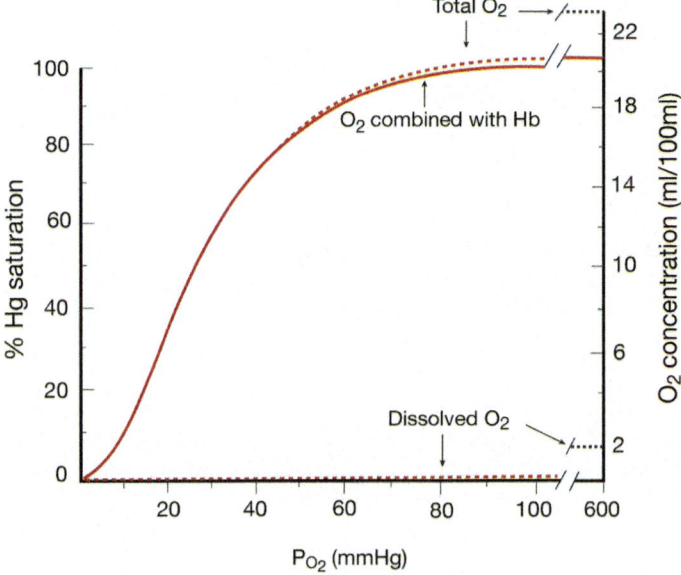

Fig. 4.8 Oxygen dissociation curve

- O_2 forms a reversible combination with Hb, with 1 g of Hb combining with 1.34 mL of O_2 → as we have around 150 g of Hb/L^{-1}, this means it can carry 201 mL/L^{-1} of oxygen (70 times more oxygen per L)
- O_2 saturation is the measurement of the proportion of oxygen being carried by haemoglobin relative to the maximal carrying capacity of haemoglobin.

$$S_{O_2} = \frac{[HbO_2]}{[Hb] \times 1.34}$$

P_{O2} of 100 mmHg → 97.5% saturation of haemoglobin
P_{O2} of 40 mmHg → 75% saturation of haemoglobin
Saturation does not take into account any underlying anaemia
Oxygen content in blood can therefore be given by (Fig. 4.8);

$$C_{O_2} = ([Hb] \times 1.34 \times S_{O_2}) + (0.03 \times P_{O_2})$$

Oxygen-Dissociation curve. This looks at the haemoglobin saturation at different partial pressures of oxygen. It is a sigmoid shape due to the co-operativity of the haemoglobin molecule (once one oxygen molecule binds, it makes it easier for the others to bind)

Flat top → Even if alveolar P_{AO2} falls somewhat → little change to the loading of Hb with oxygen

Steep descent → Peripheral tissues can withdraw large amounts of O_2 for a small change in P_{aO2}

- Cyanosis is difficult to detect in anaemic patients as approximately 50 g/L^{-1} of deoxygenated hemoglobin is needed to detect cyanosis
- **RIGHT** shift (O_2 affinity of Hb is reduced) means more unloading of O_2 at a given P_{O2}
  - ↑ in H$^+$, ↓ pH, ↑ P_{CO2}, ↑ temp, ↑ 2,3 DPG
- *IMPORTANT*: Exercising muscle is acidic, hypercarbic, and hot → It benefits from more oxygen
- **LEFT** shift (O_2 affinity of Hb is increased) favours binding of O_2
  - ↓ in H$^+$, ↑ pH, ↓ P_{CO2}, ↓ temp, ↓ 2,3 DPG, fetal Hb, CO poisoning
- 2,3 DPG produced in the glycolytic pathway, increases with hypoxic states and ↑ off loading of oxygen. Stored bank blood may be depleted of 2,3 DPG.
- P_{50} (partial pressure at which Hb is 50% saturated) is a good indicator of the curve position → normal is 27 mmHg (Fig. 4.9)
- CO_2 is carried in the blood as (1) dissolved, (2) bicarbonate, (3) carbamino compounds
  - CO_2 is about 20 times more soluble than O_2 hence a larger percentage is dissolved in blood (~10% in venous blood)
  - Bicarbonate (via carbonic acid) $CO_2 + H_2O \rightarrow H_2CO_3 \rightarrow H^+ + HCO_3^-$ (~60% in venous blood). The presence of carbonic acid enzyme in the RBC speeds up the initial hydrolysis of CO_2.
  - Carbamino compounds → CO_2 combines with terminal amine groups (~30% in venous blood) as Hb is the most abundant protein in blood, Hb contributes to the largest proportion of CO_2 carried in this form.
- CO_2 dissociation curve is much more linear and also much steeper

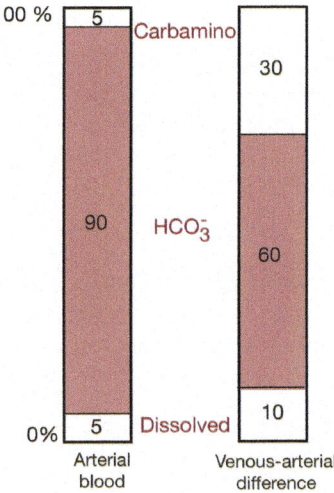

Fig. 4.9 Carbon dioxide transport

4 Respiratory Physiology

- HCO_3^- (which is negatively charged) diffuses out of the cell. In order to maintain electrical neutrality, in accordance to the Gibbs-Donnan law, Cl^- diffuses into the RBC.
- The uptake of CO_2 by the RBC, increases the osmolar concentration of the cell, hence water diffuses in also. This means the RBC increases in size in the periphery, compared to the lung.

Acid – base status

- Lung has a profound effect on acid-base balance
- pH_a is determined by the HCO_3^- / P_{aCO_2} ratio where:

$$pH_a = 6.1 + \log_{10}\left(\frac{[HCO_3^-]}{P_{aCO_2} \times 0.03}\right) \quad (6.1 = \text{dissociation constant})$$

- pH_a can be disturbed in four ways:
    - Respiratory Acidosis (↑ in P_{aCO2}, lesser ↑ in HCO_3^-, with overall ↓ in the ratio and therefore ↓ in the pH_a)
        - Caused by CO_2 retention → hypoventilation or $\dot{V}/\dot{Q}$ inequality
        - With time the kidney responds by conserving HCO_3^- → more acid urine → net compensation
    - Respiratory Alkalosis (↓P_{aCO2}, lesser ↓ in HCO_3^-, ↑ in ratio and ↑ in pH_a)
        - Caused by hyperventilation
        - Renal compensation occurs by excreting in HCO_3^- with a reduction in HCO_3^-
    - Metabolic Acidosis (↓ in HCO_3^-, lesser ↓ in P_{aCO2}, ↓ in ratio, ↓ in pH_a)
        - May be caused by diabetic ketoacidosis, lactic acid
        - Respiratory compensation is through ↑ ventilation (stimulated by chemoreceptors)
    - Metabolic Alkalosis (↑ in HCO_3^-, ~ slight ↑ in P_{aCO2}, ↑ in ratio, ↑ in pH_a)
        - Caused by ingestion of alkali

4.7 Mechanics of Breathing

Questions

1. What is the main muscle of respiration? What direction does it move in inspiration?
   Diaphragm; downwards- 1 cm in quiet respiration but up to 10 cm in deep inspiration.

2. Name the accessory muscles of inspiration?
   Scalenes and sternocleidomastoid muscles.

3. What are the muscles of expiration?
   Expiration is largely a passive phenomenon due to the elastic recoil of the lungs. However the abdominal wall muscles and *internal* intercostal muscles can aid active expiration.

4. What effect does age have on airway closure volumes?
   As age increases, the volume at which the airways closes increases (e.g. gets closer to FRC).

5. Define compliance of the lung.
   This is the volume change per unit pressure change; equates to the slope of the pressure volume curve (Fig. 4.10).

6. Name two conditions that decrease lung compliance?
   (a) Pulmonary surfactant deficiency/dysfunction
   (b) Pulmonary fibrosis
   (c) Alveolar oedema
   (d) Atelectasis
   (e) Increased venous pressure

7. Name two conditions that increase the lung compliance?
   (a) Emphysema
   (b) Age

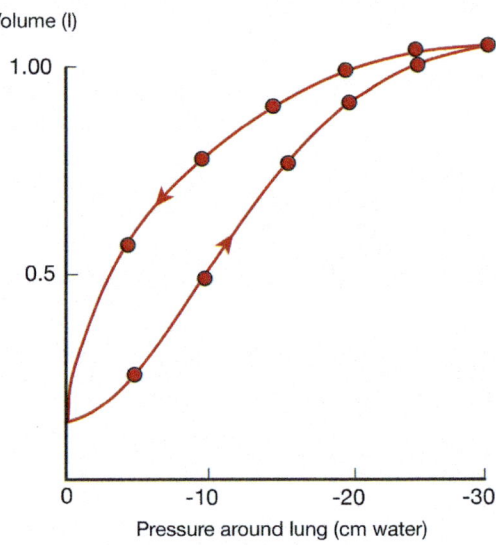

Fig. 4.10 Pressure-Volume loop

8. Describe the mechanism by which a pulmonary embolism decreases the surfactant production.
   Surfactant is produced by type 2 pneumocytes in the lungs. It is a mixture of ~95% phospholipid and 5% protein. DPPC (dipalmitoylphosphatidylcholine) is the most abundant phospholipid. This is produced from fatty acids, which are extracted from the lungs blood circulation. The turnover of surfactant is rapid, hence will be quickly depleted in the setting of decreased blood supply (e.g. a PE).

9. What role does surfactant play?

   (a) Decreases the surface tension in the alveoli hence decreases the work of breathing
   (b) Increases the stability of the alveoli
   (c) Prevents transudation of fluid

10. How does surfactant work?
    Surfactant phospholipids have hydrophobic tails and hydrophilic heads. This makes them energetically favour the surface environment in polar solvents (e.g. water). As the intermolecular attraction of phospholipids is much lower than that of water, by displacing water at the surface, the surface tension is lowered ~1/5 that of plasma.

11. What are the two types of flow through a tube?
    Laminar flow and turbulent flow.

12. In an asthmatic, bronchoconstriction halves the radius of the bronchioles. If the flow is laminar, how much is the resistance to flow increased by?
    16 times. Resistance is inversely proportional to r^4.

13. What two factors are proportional to resistance to laminar flow?
    Viscosity of the fluid and length of the tube.

14. In turbulent flow, is it viscosity or density that is more important to the resistance of flow?
    Density.

15. What equation can be used to predict if flow is going to be turbulent or laminar?
    Reynolds number.

$$\text{Re} = \frac{\rho \times u \times L}{\mu} = \frac{\text{inertial component}}{\text{viscous component}}$$

(L = linear dimension (diameter); u = velocity; ρ = density; μ = viscosity).

- If Re is <2300 then flow is likely to be laminar.
- If Re is >2300 and <4000 then flow is likely to be transitional.
- If Re is >4000 then flow is likely to be turbulent.

16. Why might heliox be used in asthma?
    This is because there is high airways resistance with turbulent flow in asthma. Heliox is a mixture of 79% helium and 21% oxygen. It has a lower density than air. This means that it lessens the resistance to turbulent flow and delivers more gas to the alveoli.

Short notes

- Primary muscle of inspiration is the diaphragm; usually moves about 1 cm but may move up to 10 cm in deep inspiration
    - If paralysed may move paradoxically (e.g. phrenic nerve palsy)
    - External intercostal muscles play a much smaller role in changing the anterior-posterior diameter
- Expiration is usually passive, but, if active, is primarily through the abdominal wall muscles assisted by the internal intercostal muscles.
    The curve the lung follows for inflation and deflation are different → this is known as hysteresis (Fig. 4.10).
    - The lung volume at any given pressure is greater during deflation (airways may be held open)
- Compliance is the slope in the pressure volume curve.
    - In the normal range the lung is very compliant, at higher pressures it flattens off (*see* Fig. 4.10)
    - Reduced compliance is caused by fibrotic tissue, atelectasis and blood engorgement
    - Increased compliance occurs with emphysema and normal aging (↓ elastic tissue)
- Surface tension plays an important role in lung compliance (reduces compliance as it hold surfaces together).
    - Surfactant significantly lowers the surface tension and stabilises the alveoli (especially at small volumes) and keeps them dry
    - Produced by type 2 pneumocytes
- Intrapleural pressure is less negative at the bottom of the lung than at the top of the lung.
    - Lung is easier to inflate at lower volumes than higher volumes
    - Expanding pressure at the base is small due to a smaller resting volume making it easier to expand
    - Expanding pressure at the apex is large due to a larger resting volume making it more difficult to expand
    - With aging, airway closure with trapping may occur at relatively normal pressures as the closing volumes reach the FRC (Fig. 4.11)

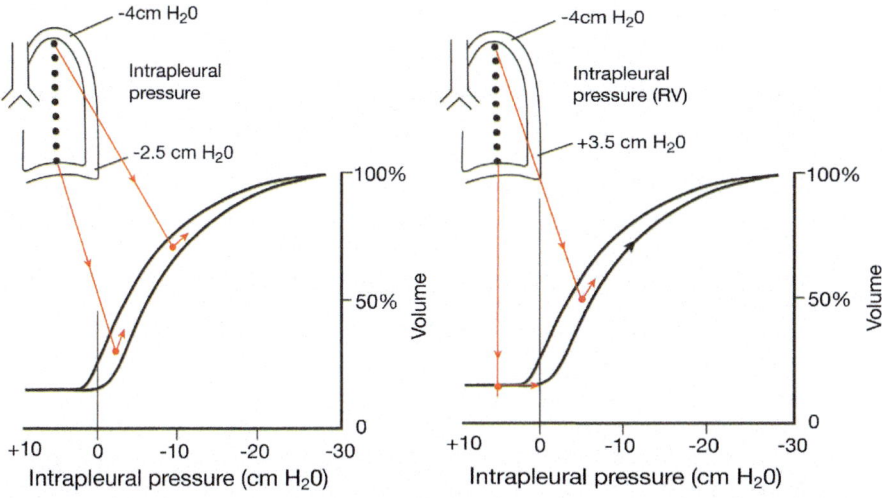

Fig. 4.11 Compliance at different intrapleural pressures

- The chest wall has a tendency to spring out and the lung has a tendency to collapse inwards.
  - These tendencies normally create a small negative intrapleural pressure
  - The FRC is the point at which the want of the chest wall to spring out and the lung to recoil is balanced, and the airway pressure is 0
  - The lung wants to recoil at all volumes, the chest wall wants to spring out until 75% of VC

Flow:
Laminar flow rate depends on (1) Δ pressure (2) radius^4, (3) viscosity and (4) length. Therefore the resistance to laminar flow is calculated by;

$$\text{Re} = \frac{8 \times \mu \times l}{\pi \times r^4}$$

(μ = viscosity; l = length; r = radius)

Turbulent flow is more dependent on density and less on viscosity. There is more resistance to turbulent flow and hence a greater driving pressure is needed. Whether flow will be laminar or turbulent depends on Reynolds number;

$$\text{Re} = \frac{\rho \times u \times L}{\mu} = \frac{\text{inertial component}}{\text{viscous component}}$$

(L = linear dimention (diameter); u = velocity; ρ = density; μ = viscosity).

Flow type	Laminar	Transitional	Turbulent
Reynolds number	<2300	>2300 and <4000	>4000

Reynolds number is low in the terminal bronchioles but higher in the trachea, especially during exercise.

- Airway resistance can be calculated from the pressure difference divided by the flow rate
- In inspiration, the pressure change to promote flow is generally very small (1 cmH$_2$O) but in airway obstruction it can be many times this
- Major site of resistance is in the medium sized airways (up to the 7th generation)
- Bronchi are supported by radial traction
    - As lung volumes reduce, airway resistance is increased dramatically, with small airways closing completely at the bottom of the lung
    - Patients with ↑ airway resistance breathe at higher lung volumes → this ↓ the resistance
    - Smooth muscle contraction (irritants, parasympathetic response) significantly increases resistance
- The expiratory flow rate is independent of effort. This is due to dynamic airway compression. In forced expiration the intrapleural pressure becomes greater than the pressure in the airway and causes compression of the airway which may result in air trapping.
- Uneven ventilation can be caused by local variations in compliance and resistance and resulting in heterogeneous distribution of ventilation, this may cause some regions of the lung to have higher or lower P$_{O2}$ and P$_{CO2}$.
- Work of breathing can best be defined as pressure × volume
    - Work is expended to overcome elastic tissue forces and viscous airway forces
    - Energy invested in overcoming tissue forces allows for passive expiration

Overall efficiency of breathing is about 5–10%, O$_2$ cost of quiet breathing is about 5% of the total resting oxygen consumption (Fig. 4.12).

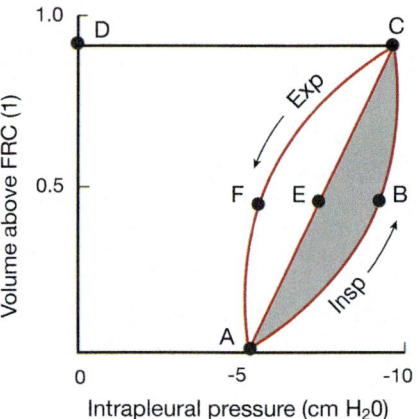

Fig. 4.12 Work of breathing

4 Respiratory Physiology

4.8 Control of Ventilation

Questions

1. Which sensors are the most important for minute to minute control of ventilation?
   The chemoreceptors near the ventral surface of the medulla in the vicinity of the 9th and 10th cranial nerve site of exit.

2. What is the main driver of central chemoreceptors?
   H^+ ions. (*see short notes*).

3. What is the normal pH of CSF.
   pH = 7.32; the CSF has less ability to buffer changes in pH compared to blood.

4. Where are peripheral chemoreceptors located?
   In the carotid bodies at the bifurcation of the common carotid arteries and in the aortic bodies above and below the arch. In humans the carotid bodies are the most important.

5. What do the peripheral chemoreceptors respond to?
   Decreased P_{aO2}, pH and increased P_{aCO2}.

6. Why can you hold your breath for longer if you hyperventilate first?
   Hyperventilation reduces P_{aCO2} and hence C_{aCO2}. As the relative carrying capacity for CO_2 is much greater than that of O_2, the time taken for P_{aCO2} to rise to a level to significantly contribute to respiratory drive is greater.

7. Why do some patients with COPD rely heavily on their peripheral chemoreceptors response to lower P_{aO2}?
   This is because they have chronically raised levels of CO_2 in the blood. Overtime there is equilibration of the ECF in the brain, so despite high P_{aCO2}, the pH is normal. Under these situations, arterial hypoxaemia is the biggest drive for ventilation (i.e. type II respiratory failure).

8. What are the main drivers of ventilation in exercise?
   The mechanism for control of ventilation during exercise is not fully understood, however it is likely to be as a consequence of a number of feedforward and feedback mechanisms with the involvement of mechano-receptors, chemo-receptors and possibly thermo-receptors. This mechanism maintains P_{aCO2} and P_{aO2} across a wide range of workload and these parameters are only disturbed when physiological limitations to aerobic exercise are reached.

Short notes

1. The three basic elements of respiratory control at rest are sensors, central controllers and effectors, usually operating in a negative feedback fashion
2. Central Control
   (a) Control of breathing is in the brainstem (pons and medulla)

(b) Can be voluntarily overridden by the cortex

- Medullary respiratory centre (reticular formation of the medulla)
  - Dorsal respiratory group controls inspiration – thought to have intrinsic firing properties
  - Ventral respiratory group controls expiration – usually quiescent during normal breathing
- Apneustic centre (lower pons)
- Pneumotaxic centre (upper pons) appears to switch off the medullary respiratory centre

(c) Cortex can halve P_{aCO2} with hyperventilation and also cause significant hypoventilation

(d) The limbic system and hypothalamus can further alter breathing

3. Effectors

    (a) Important that these are coordinated

4. Sensors (Fig. 4.13)

    (a) Central – *most important for minute to minute ventilation*

    - Located on the ventral surface of the medulla (~200–400 mm below ventral surface of medulla)
    - Surrounded by brain ECF and responds to $\Delta[H^+]$; stimulates ventilation and vice versa
    - ECF composition is determined by CSF, local blood flow and local metabolism
    - Mechanism is $\uparrow P_{aCO2} \rightarrow$ vasodilation $\rightarrow CO_2$ diffuses to the CSF $\rightarrow$ liberates $H^+ \rightarrow$ alters pH
      - Note that CSF pH has less ability to be buffered than normal blood
      - This system normalises in the long term and can lead to CO_2 retention

    (b) Peripheral

    - Located in the carotid bodies at the bifurcation of the common carotid artery and the aortic bodies above and below the aortic arch. Carotid bodies are more important in humans.
      - Respond to P_{aO2}, $\downarrow pH_a$ and $\uparrow$ in P_{aCO2}
      - Response to mild decreases in P_{aO2} is small, in most individuals significant increases in ventilation as a consequence of hypoxia only occurs when $P_{aO2} < 70$ mmHg.
      - Responsible for ventilatory changes in relation to arterial hypoxemia
      - Carotid receptors respond to Δ pH and potentiates the hypoxic response
      - Response to P_{aCO2} is less important but also potentiates the hypoxic response

Fig. 4.13 Central chemoreceptor

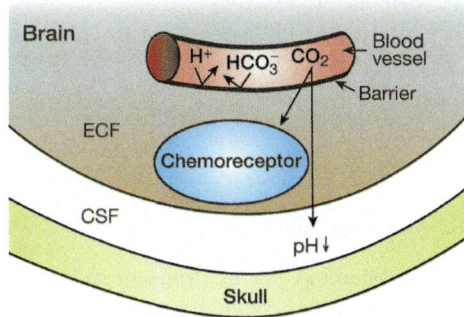

- Lung Receptors
    - Pulmonary stretch receptors lie in the airway smooth muscle
    - Irritant receptors lie between the airway epithelial cells and impulses travel via the vagus nerve → bronchoconstriction and hyperpnea
    - J–receptors (juxta-capillary) hypothesised to be in the alveolar walls close to capillaries resulting in rapid shallow breathing with engorgement
    - Bronchial C fibres – respond to chemical changes in the bronchial (not pulmonary) circulation
- Other
    - Nose, pharynx and trachea receptors respond to stimulation
- Joint and muscle receptors are believed to stimulate ventilation
- Gamma system – respiratory muscles contain muscle spindles which reflexly controls the strength of contraction
- Arterial baroreceptors – increased arterial blood pressure can cause hypoventilation through stimulation of aortic or carotid sinus baroreceptors
- Pain and temperature

5. Response to carbon dioxide
    (a) Ventilation is closely controlled to maintain P_{aCO2}
    (b) Both central and peripheral chemoreceptors mediate the response to changes in P_{aCO2}
    (c) A reduction in P_{aCO2} can reduce the stimulus to ventilate
    (d) Response is reduced by sleep, age, drugs (opioids) and other factors

6. Response to oxygen
    (a) If P_{aCO2} is unchanged, P_{aO2} can drop to about 50 mmHg before a significant effect is noticed
    (b) In P_{aCO2} retention (type II respiratory failure) the hypoxic drive is very important. In this situation increasing P_{aO2} with supplementary oxygen may cause hypoventilation resulting in severe respiratory acidosis and such patients need to be closely monitored

7. Response to exercise
   (a) Ventilation may increase by up to 15 times, with all of the exact factors largely unknown. Albeit the mechanism for control of ventilation during exercise is not fully understood, however it is likely to be as a consequence of a number of feedforward and feedback mechanisms with the involvement of mechano-receptors, chemo-receptors and possibly thermo-receptors
8. Abnormal breathing
   (a) Seen in Cheyne Stokes breathing with significant fluctuation most likely due to cardiac resynchronization with the respiratory drive.
   (b) Seen in brain damage, heart disease and increased altitude

Chapter 5
Renal Physiology

S. Ali Mirjalili, Lucy Hinton, and Kevin Ellyett

5.1 Body Water

Questions

1. Under normal conditions, by which route is the most water lost from the body?
   Urine.
   Urine (500 mL/day to 20 L/day)
   Insensible 700 mL/day (skin 300–400, respiratory 300–400 mL/day)
   Sweat (Variable)
   Faeces ~200 mL/day.

2. What percentage of total body weight is water in a 70 kg male?
   60%.

3. What are the different fluid compartments in the body? What ratio of total body water do they make up?
   Intracellular fluid (ICF) – 2/3
   Extracellular fluid (ECF) – 1/3 (1/4 plasma, 3/4 interstitial fluid)

4. What is the transcellular fluid compartment?
   Transcellular compartment is the component of extracellular water that lies within epithelial lined spaces e.g. pleura, pericardium. It is around 1–2 L.

S. A. Mirjalili (✉)
Department of Anatomy and Medical Imaging, University of Auckland, Auckland, New Zealand
e-mail: a.mirjalili@auckland.ac.nz

L. Hinton
Department of General Surgery, Tauranga Hospital, Tauranga, New Zealand

K. Ellyett
University of Auckland, Auckland, New Zealand

Auckland Hospital, Auckland, New Zealand

Daily Intake and Output of Water (ml/day)

	Normal	Prolonged Heavy Exercise
Intake		
Fluids ingested	2100	?
From metabolism	200	200
Total intake	2300	?
Output		
Insensible - skin	350	350
Insensible - lungs	350	650
Sweat	100	5000
Feces	100	100
Urine	1400	500
Total output	2300	6600

Fig. 5.1 Water balance

5. Does total body water vary proportionally or is it inversely proportional to fat?
   Inversely proportional.
   This is why women have a lower total body water percentage than men (55% vs 60%)

6. In regards to the ECF compartment; is the protein concentration greater in the interstitial fluid or the plasma?
   The protein concentration is higher in the plasma. This is because the capillaries have a low permeability to the plasma proteins.

7. What ions have the highest concentration in the ICF and ECF?
   Intracellular- Potassium and Phosphate
   Extracellular- Sodium and Chloride

8. How can intracellular fluid volume be calculated?
   It cannot be measured directly.
   It can be derived by measuring the volume of total body water and subtracting the volume of the extracellular fluid.

Total body water

The regulation of body water is one of the key functions of the kidneys. This is maintained tightly despite large variations in water gain and loss (Fig. 5.1).

Gain

1. Ingestion ~2000 mL/day
2. Metabolism 200 mL/day

Loss

1. Insensible 700 mL/day (skin 300–400 mL, respiratory 300–400 mL/day)
2. Sweat (Variable)
3. Faeces ~200 mL/day.
4. Urine (500 mL/day to 20 L/day)

Overall, water is 60% of total body weight (42 L).

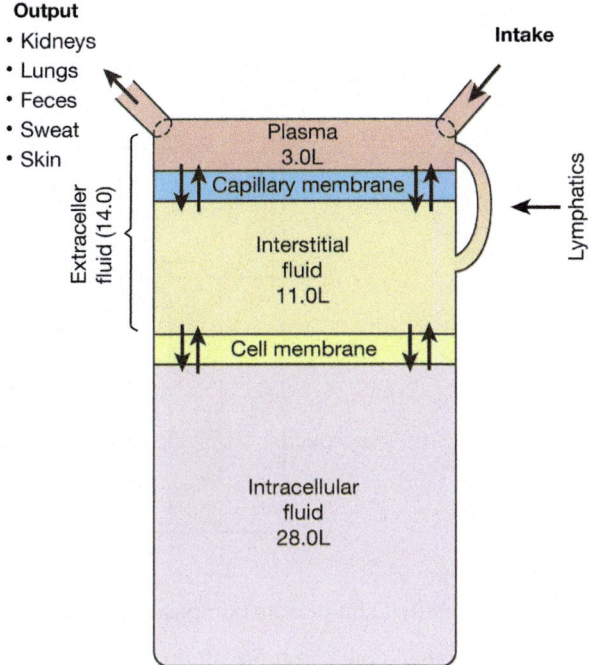

Fig. 5.2 Water in body compartments

There are different fluid compartments (Fig. 5.2):

- 2/3 is intracellular (28 L).
- 1/3 is extracellular (14 L); of which 1/4 is plasma (3 L) and 3/4 is interstitial fluid (9 L).
- Transcellular compartment (1–2 L) is the portion of total body water contained within epithelial lined spaces e.g. pleura, pericardium.
- Adipose tissue has less water than muscle + other tissues high in protein. Therefore women, elderly and obese have decreased percentage of body water as they have a higher proportion of adipose tissue.
- There are different compositions of ions in the different body compartments (Fig. 5.3).

Difference between ICF and ECF;

- ICF contains a high amount of K^+ (160 mmol/L) and PO_4^{-3} (130 mmol/L)
- ECF contains a high amount of Na^+, Cl^- and HCO_3^-
- Total exchangeable sodium in the body is approximately 3000 mmol, this being 70% of the total body Na^+. The total body K^+ is approximately 3000 mmol and of this, 90% is exchangeable.

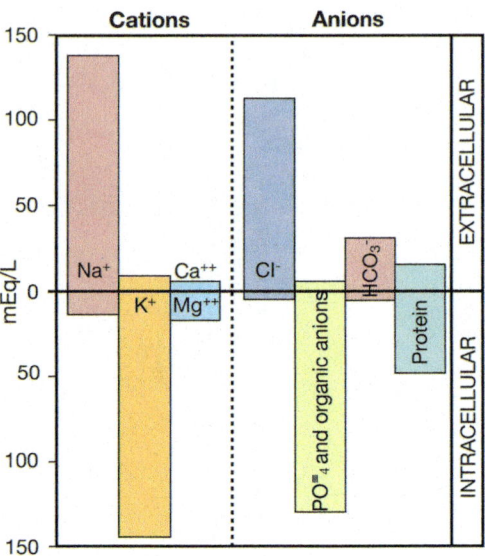

Fig. 5.3 Ionic concentrations

Difference between interstitial and plasma composition of ECF;

- Plasma has a higher concentration of proteins, which are negatively charged, than the interstitial fluid.
- Therefore plasma has more cations (which are attracted to the negatively charged proteins) and interstitial fluid has more anions.

Measurement of compartments:
What is used to measure the different compartments volumes;

- Total body water: Radioactive water, deuterium oxide dilution
- ECF: Radioactive Na^+, radioactive Cl^-, Inulin
- ICF: Cannot be measured directly = Calculated from TBW − ECF
- Plasma: Radioactive albumin
- Interstitial fluid: Cannot be measured directly = Calculated from ECF − Plasma

Total body osmolarity is ~300 mOsm/L. Solutions can be isotonic, hypotonic (cause the cells to swell), hypertonic (cause the cells to shrink).

5.2 Function of Glomerulus and Tubules

1. What are the three ways that solutes can be handled in the glomerulus and the tubules?

    (a) Filtered
    (b) Reabsorbed
    (c) Secreted

5 Renal Physiology

2. What percentage of the filtered load of water is reabsorbed in the proximal tubule?
   ~70%.
   The GFR is 125 mL/min, this means that 180 L of water is filtered a day. 70% of this is reabsorbed in the proximal tubule.

3. What is the most important carrier protein in the ascending limb of the Loop of Henle?
   NaK2Cl.
   This is powered by secondary active transport. The basolateral Na/K ATPase decreases the intracellular concentration of Na^+. This allows for the Na^+ to diffuse out of the tubular fluid down its concentration gradient. It carries the other ions with it as it does so.
   This is blocked by Frusemide.

4. What part of the Loop of Henle is permeable to water?
   The thin descending portion.
   The ascending potion is then impermeable to water and permeable to ions (via the NaK2Cl channel). This aids the creation of the high medullary concentration.

5. What is the most important transport protein in the distal convoluted tubule?
   It is the NaCl co-transporter.
   This is powered by the basolateral Na/K ATPase, which sets up a concentration gradient for Na^+. This allows Na^+ and Cl^- transport through the luminal aspect via the NaCl co transporter.
   This is blocked by thiazide diuretics.

6. What is the function of the intercalated cells of the distal and collecting tubules?
   Intercalated cells reabsorb K^+ ions and HCO_3^- while secreting H^+ ions. The H^+ is secreted by the H^+ ATPase (plays an integral part of acid regulation).

7. Which cell does Aldosterone act on?
   The principal cells of the distal tubule and collecting duct.

The Glomerulus (Fig. 5.4)
Glomerulus and Bowman's capsule- The glomerulus has a unique arrangement; the capillary bed lies between two arterioles (the afferent and efferent arteriole). This allows for control of the filtration pressure. It is here that the ultra filtrate is produced and is filtered into the Bowman's capsule.

Proximal tubule
Anatomy: Lined by columnar epithelium with tight junctions between them, luminal surface area increased by the presence of brush border microvilli. They have a high number of mitochondria due to their high metabolic rate.
Function: Receive 180 L/day of glomerular filtrate, reabsorb approximately 70% (127 L/day).
The most important substances to be reabsorbed in the proximal tubules are Na^+ (65% of filtered load), HCO_3^- (~85% of filtered load), Cl^- (~65% of filtered load), glucose (100% of filtered load, under normal conditions) and water.

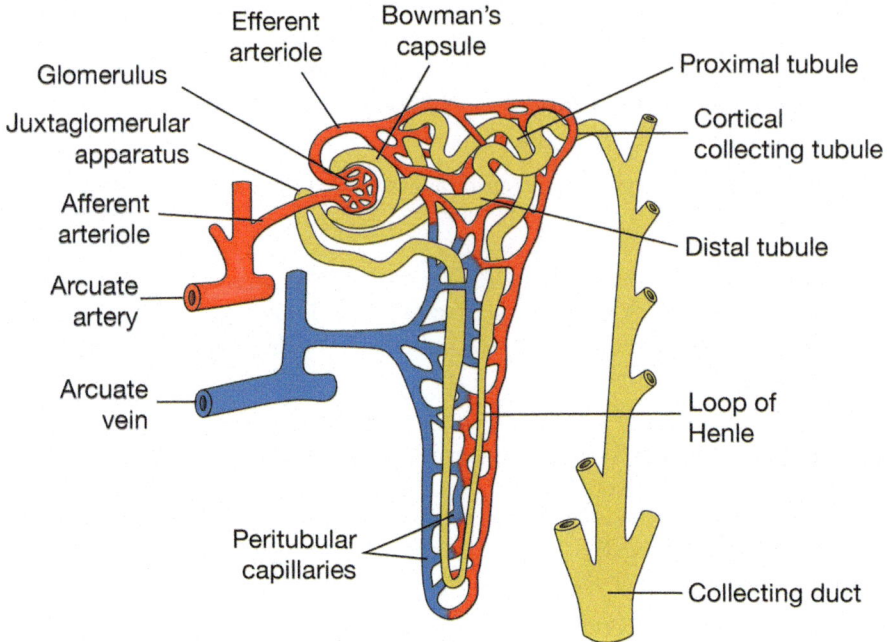

Fig. 5.4 The Nephron

The proximal tubule is also able to secrete certain substances, such an organic acids and bases into the lumen for excretion in the urine.

The osmolarity stays the same along the PCT as water is absorbed along with the solutes.

Loop of Henle

Anatomy: The Loop of Henle (LoH) descends from the renal cortex as the descending limb and then does a U-turn to become the ascending limb. It can be divided into three functional parts- thin descending, thin ascending and thick ascending portion. There are two types of LoH; cortical (85%) and juxtamedullary (15%) depending on how far they descend into the medulla.

Function: Of the original 180 L/day filtered at the glomerulus, 30 L is reabsorbed in the descending limb of the Loop of Henle.

Main function of the LoH is to form a high osmotic concentration in the renal medulla, which allows for the absorption of water from the collecting ducts.

Thin descending – permeable to water, relatively impermeable to ions.

Ascending – Permeable to ions via the NaK2Cl transporter, impermeable to water. 25% of the filtered loads of Na^+, Cl^-, and K^+ are reabsorbed in the Loop of Henle, mostly in the thick ascending limb.

Channels: NaK2Cl and Na/H antiporter on the luminal aspect.

Secondary active transport is powered by basolateral Na/K ATPase; decreases intracellular Na^+ concentration, sets up concentration gradient for diffusion of Na^+. Na/H counter-transport in the thick ascending limb allows for Na^+ reabsorption and H^+ secretion.

Distal Convoluted Tubule and Collecting Tubule
Anatomy: Closely associated with the macula densa, which is part of the tubuloglomerular feedback pathway.
The late distal tubule and collecting tubule are lined by two cells, the intercalated and principal cells.

Function: Variable reabsorption; Depending on Extracellular fluid volume and osmolarity- helps to 'fine tune' absorption.
Impermeable to water and urea
Varying permeability to Na^+ and Cl^-.

Channels: NaCl co-transporter.
Basolateral Na/K ATPase sets up a concentration gradient for Na^+ to diffuse down its concentration gradient via the luminal NaCl co-transporter.
Principal cells reabsorb Na^+ and water from the lumen and secrete K^+, under the influence of aldosterone.
Intercalated cells reabsorb K^+ and HCO_3^- while secreting H^+. The H^+ is secreted by the H^+ATPase (plays an integral part of acid regulation as able to secrete H^+ against a large gradient).

Collecting Duct
Anatomy: The collecting tubules coalesce to form collecting ducts. They are lined by nearly cuboid shaped cells with few mitochondria.
Divided into two regions; cortical and medullary.
They all pass through the renal cortex and medulla to empty into the pelvis of the kidney at the apexes of the medullary pyramids.

Function: Extremely important role in determining the final urine output of water and solutes.
There are several hormones that act on the collecting ducts, but the two most important are anti-diuretic hormone (ADH) and aldosterone.
Water handling is dependent on the presence of ADH.
High ADH, high water reabsorption
Low ADH, low water reabsorption
Collecting ducts are also permeable to urea, this helps to raise the osmolarity in the medulla.

5.3 Renal Blood Flow

1. What principle can be applied when measuring renal blood flow (RBF)?
   Fick's principle. This is equal to the amount of the substance taken up per unit time divided by the arterio-venous difference.

2. What substance is used to calculate RBF, why is this substance used?
   Para-aminohippuric acid. This is used as it is filtered at the glomerulus and then secreted into the tubule, but not reabsorbed.

3. What effect does noradrenaline have on renal blood flow?
   It decreases RBF. It constricts both the afferent and efferent arterioles.

4. Where is the macula densa found?
   This is found at the confluence of the thick ascending limb of Loop of Henle and DCT. It lies in close proximity to the afferent arteriole (Fig. 5.5).

5. How does Tubuloglomerular feedback work to alter RBF?
   This helps to auto regulate the delivery of blood to the glomerulus, based upon the composition of the filtrate reaching the DCT.
   In situations of high Na$^+$ (and water) in the tubular fluid, the macula densa, located in the distal convoluted tubule, will absorb Na$^+$ through the luminal NaK2Cl channel. This is then pumped out of the basolateral side by the Na/K ATPase, in doing so adenosine is produced. The adenosine then binds to the adenosine A1 receptor on the afferent arteriole. This increases the intracellular concentration of

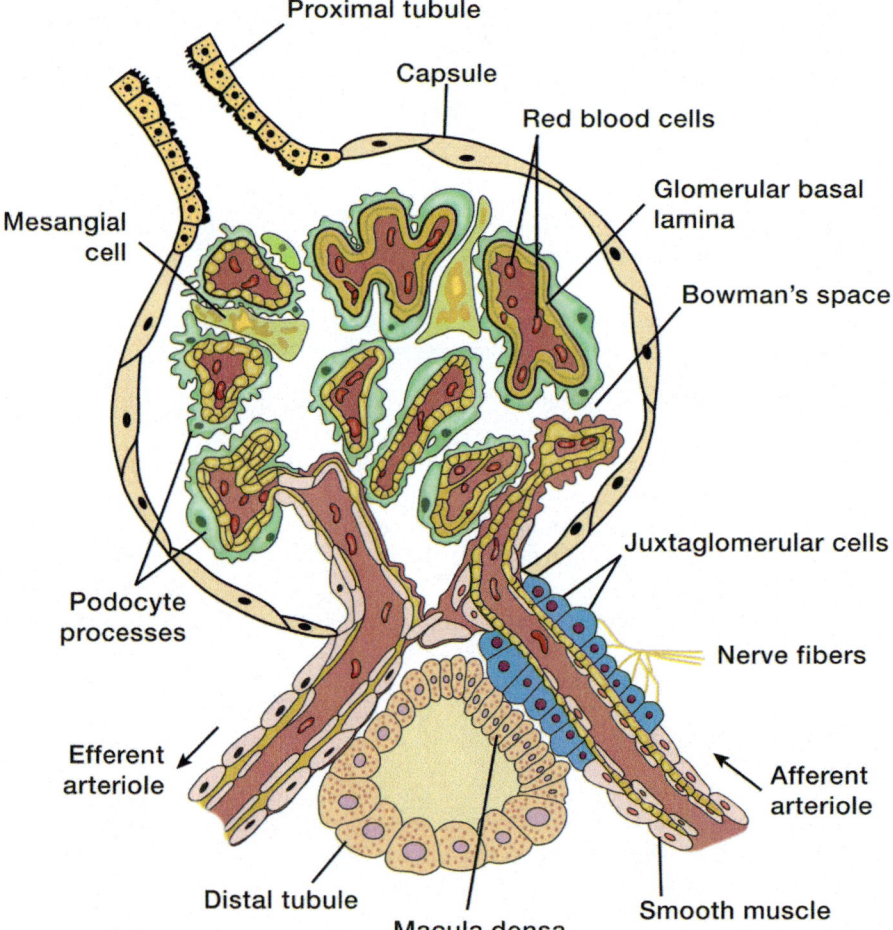

Fig. 5.5 Cross section of the glomerulus and Bowman's capsule

Ca²⁺ and causes vasoconstriction, therefore decreasing the RBF. The converse is true when there is a low concentration of Na⁺ reaching the DCT.

6. Using Fick's principle, what is used to calculate GFR?
Inulin. This is because it is freely filtered in the glomerulus, but not secreted or reabsorbed.

7. Why is Creatinine used to calculate the eGFR?
This is because it is an endogenous product, produced during muscle metabolism. Unlike inulin, it is secreted into the tubules, so using it to calculate the eGFR will slightly overestimate the eGFR.

8. What are the determinants of the GFR?

$$GFR = Kf\left[(P_{GC} - P_T) - (\pi_{GC} - \pi_T)\right]$$

Kf = glomerular ultra filtration coefficient
P_{GC} = mean hydrostatic pressure in the glomerular capillaries
P_T = mean hydrostatic pressure in the tubule (Bowman's space)
π_{GC} = oncotic pressure of the plasma in the glomerular capillaries
π_T = oncotic pressure in the filtrate of the tubule

The kidneys are well set up for filtration as they have high Kf and a high hydrostatic pressure as the capillaries lie between two arterioles.

The RBF and GFR

Renal blood flow = 20% of CO, which equates to 1250 mL/min. High blood flow to be able to maintain the filtration rate.
Renal clearance = Volume of plasma cleared of a substance by the kidneys per unit time. Depending on how the substance is handled by the kidney depends on what renal clearance measures.
Clearance is calculated using the Fick principle:

$$Clearance = \frac{Rate\ of\ Urinary\ Excretion}{Arterial\ Plasma\ Concentration}$$

$$= \frac{Urine\ Production\ Rate \times Urine\ Concentration}{Arterial\ Plasma\ Concentration}$$

Renal Blood Flow (Fig. 5.6)

Measured using **para-aminohippuric acid** (PAH) clearance. This is a substance that is both *filtered* and *secreted* in the glomerulus, but not reabsorbed.
Auto regulation of RBF between MABP 75–170 mmHg
This is due to myogenic control and tubuloglomerular feedback.

1. Myogenic- Afferent arterioles change size based on the perfusion pressure
2. Tubuloglomerular feedback (TGF) (Fig. 5.5)

The sensing organ for TGF is the macula densa. This is located at the confluence of the thick ascending Loop of Henle and the distal convoluted tubule.

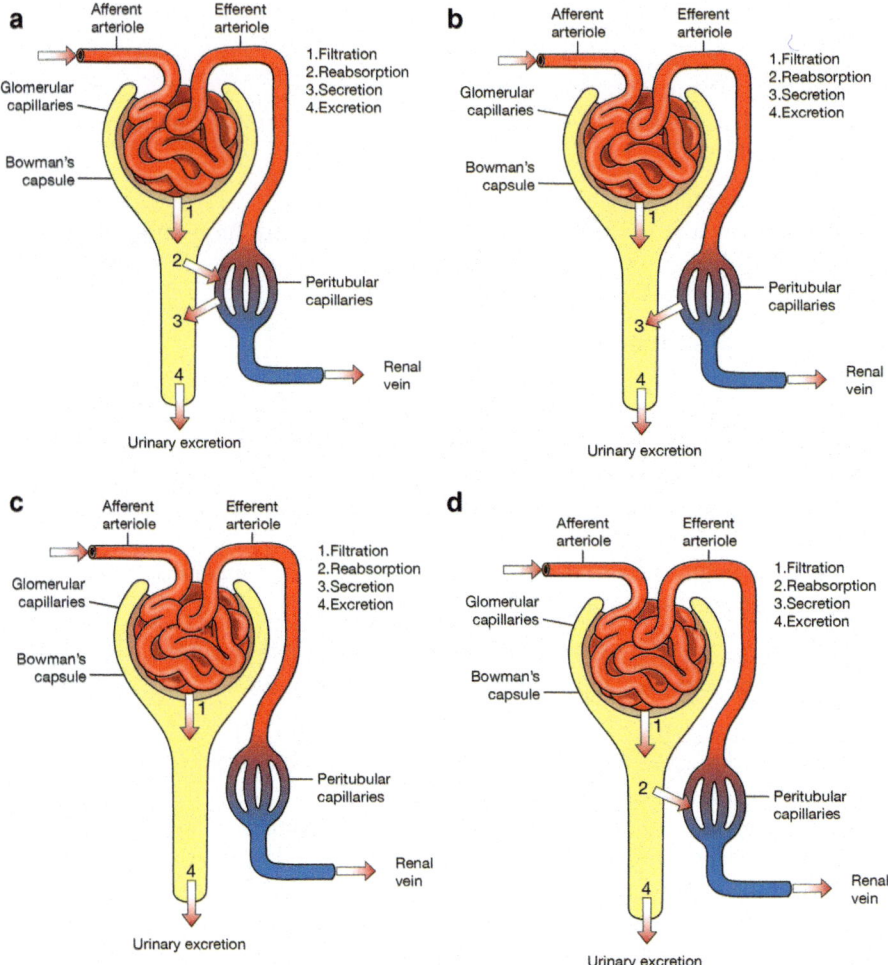

Fig. 5.6 (a) Renal handling of difference substance, (b) showing the combination of filtration, (c) reabsorption and (d) secretion

A	B	C	D
1. Filtration	PAH	Inulin	Sodium
2. Reabsorption		Freely filtered neither reabsorbed nor secreted	Reabsobed
3. Secretion	Secreted	Clearance = GFR	
4. Urinary excretion			

5 Renal Physiology

When there is high RBF, relatively more Na⁺ is filtered, which means there is more Na⁺ reaching the DCT. This is absorbed through the tubular membrane of the macula densa via the NaK2Cl transporter. This upregulates the basolateral Na/K ATPase, as it encourages the movement of Na⁺ out of the cell. In doing so, it produces more adenosine.

Adenosine drifts out of the cells and binds to adenosine A1 receptor on the afferent arterioles. This increases the intracellular Ca^{2+} concentration and causes contraction, therefore decreasing the afferent arteriole size. The converse is true when there is low RBF.

Regulation:

Noradrenaline	→ Vasoconstriction → ↓RBF
Dopamine	→ Vasodilation + natriuresis → ↑ RBF
Angiotensin II	→ Vasoconstrictor effect on both the afferent and efferent arterioles
Prostaglandins	→ ↑ blood flow in the renal cortex + ↓blood flow in the renal medulla
Acetylcholine	→ Vasodilation → ↑ RBF
High-protein diet	→ ↑ glomerular capillary pressure → ↑ RBF
Prostacyclin (PGI2)	→ Vasodilation afferent arteriole → ↑ RBF

Glomerular filtration rate

Glomerular filtration rate = Volume of fluid filtered from the glomerular capillaries into the Bowman's capsule per unit time.

Normal GFR is 125 mL/min = 180 L/day

Measured using **Inulin clearance**. This is a substance that it *filtered* but not secreted or reabsorbed.

In clinical practice, Creatinine is used. This is used as; it is an endogenous product of muscle metabolism + it has relatively steady production. This is filtered in the glomerulus, but also a small amount of secreted, so the eGFR is slightly overestimated.

Determinants of the GFR.

Like with flow through all capillaries, the GFR depends on the 'leakiness' of the capillary as well as the difference between the hydrostatic and oncotic pressure on either side of the glomerulus (Fig. 5.7).

$$GFR = Kf\left[(PGC-PT)-(\pi GC - \pi T)\right]$$

Kf = Glomerular ultra filtration coefficient. This takes into account the capillary permeability and the effective filtration surface area. The kidney has a large Kf, to allow the ultrafiltrate to be formed. Kf can be altered by contraction and relaxation of the mesangial cells (Fig. 5.8).

P_{GC} = Mean hydrostatic pressure in the glomerular capillaries. The pressure in the glomerular capillaries is higher than that in other capillary beds because the capillaries lie between two arterioles. This is usually 45 mmHg. This is what allows for the driving force of filtration. It can be manipulated to change the GFR.

Fig. 5.7 Factors affecting filtration

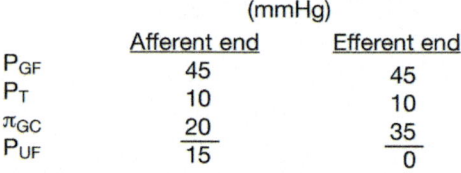

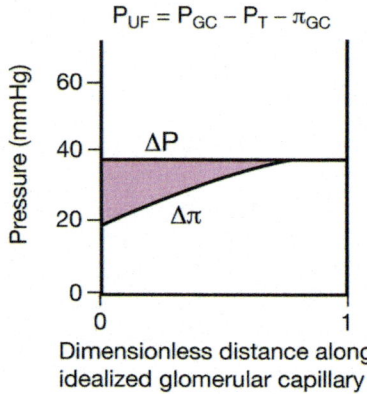

Fig. 5.8 Mesangial cells manipulating factors

Agents causing contraction or relaxation of mesangial cells

Contraction	Relaxation
Endothelins	ANP
Angiotensin II	Dopamine
Vasopressin	PGE_2
Norepinephrine	cAMP
Platelet-activating factor	
Platelet-derived growth factor	
Thromboxane A_2	
PGF_2	
Leukotrienes C_4 and D_4	
Histamine	

P_T = Mean hydrostatic pressure in the tubule (Bowman's space). This is normally 10 mmHg.

π_{GC} = Oncotic pressure of the plasma in the glomerular capillaries. This rises throughout the glomerulus. This is because plasma proteins are not easily filtered so their concentration rises throughout the glomerulus; as does the oncotic pressure. This is why there is no filtration at the end of the glomerulus (see Fig. 5.7)

5 Renal Physiology

π_T = Oncotic pressure of the filtrate in the tubule (Bowman's space). Normally negligible.

The net filtration pressure (P_{UF}) is 15 mmHg at the afferent end of the glomerular capillaries, but it falls to zero—that is, filtration equilibrium is reached—proximal to the efferent end of the glomerular capillaries. This is because fluid leaves the plasma whereas the plasma proteins do not and the oncotic pressure rises.

The ability of individual molecules to be filtered depends on their molecular weight and charge.

Molecular weight

<7000 Daltons	Molecules will be freely filtered
>70 000 Daltons	Molecules are essentially not filtered at all
7000–70,000 Daltons	Percentage of a given molecule that is filtered decreases with increasing molecular weight

Electrical charge

The sialoprotein proteins in the glomerular basement membrane proteins are negatively charged. This means that for products with molecular weights between 7000 and 70,000 Daltons, positively charged molecules will be filtered more freely than those that are negatively charged. This is why albumin, which is less than 70,000 Daltons is not filtered at the glomerulus, as it is negatively charged.

5.4 Control of Osmolarity, ECF and RBF

Questions

1. What two stimuli are the most important factors leading to release of aldosterone from the adrenal cortex?
   Hyperkalaemia and Angiotensin II.

2. Where in the kidney does Aldosterone act?
   It works in the DCT + CT. It increases the activity of Na/K ATPase on the basolateral side as well as the luminal transport of Na, through insertion of eNaC channels. It acts to increase the reabsorption of Na^+ and the secretion of K^+ and H^+.

3. What is the range of urine osmolarity?
   50–1200 mOsm/L. This is dependent on the presence of ADH.

4. Where is renin released from?
   Renin is released from the granular cells in the juxtaglomerular apparatus near the afferent arteriole. It is released in response to decreased arteriolar wall tension, SNS stimulation and decreased Na^+ or Cl^-.

5. What does anti-diuretic hormone (ADH) do?
   It allows for the reabsorption of water in the late distal tubules, collecting tubules, and collecting ducts. ADH binds to specific V2 receptors and increases the number of aquaporin-2 (AQP-2) in the luminal cell membrane. The molecules of AQP-2, which are found in intracellular vesicles, cluster together and fuse with

the cell membrane by exocytosis. They form water channels that permit rapid diffusion of water through the cells.

6. How does Frusemide work?
It is a loop diuretic which prevents the action of NaK2Cl in the LoH.

Control of RBF and GFR

Sympathetic nervous system
This acts to decrease the RBF, but conserved GFR.

NA released from the SNS, binds to α1 adrenoreceptors to cause vasoconstriction of both the afferent and efferent arterioles. This results in a significantly reduced renal blood flow. However, glomerular perfusion pressure is maintained due to greater constriction of the efferent arterioles. Overall the GFR only drops a small amount.

Renin-Angiotensin-Aldosterone system

1. Renin — This is secreted from the 'granular' cells in response to decreased afferent arteriole wall tension, SNS activity acting on β1 adrenoreceptors, prostaglandins or decreased Na^+ and Cl^- delivery to the macula densa. This is released in the blood stream.
2. Angiotensinogen – Renin is an enzyme, which converts angiotensinogen to angiotensin I.
3. Angiotensin I – In the lungs angiotensin I is converted to angiotensin II by angiotensin converting enzyme (ACE)
4. Angiotensin II – is the body's most powerful Na^+ reabsorbing hormone.
It has multiple effects; ↑ ADH release from posterior pituitary, potent vasoconstriction of BV (efferent > afferent arterioles), facilitates release of noradrenaline from sympathetic neurons, ↑ water intake by acting on the subfornical organ, directly stimulates Na^+ reabsorption in PT, LoH, DCT and CD, by direct effect on the Na/K ATPase as well as Na/H exchange in the proximal tubule.
5. Aldosterone – Secreted from the zona glomerulosa of the adrenal cortex in response to ↑ $[K^+]$ in ECF, ↑ATII, ↓ $[Na^+]$ and ACTH from anterior pituitary.

$[K^+]$ and ATII are the most important factors.
Aldosterone acts on the principal cells. It is a steroid hormone so it diffuses into the cells → binds to the cytoplasmic mineralocorticoid receptor → moves into the nucleus → forms mRNA.
Two effects;

1. ↑ production of Na/K ATPase, which are inserted into the basolateral membrane
2. ↑ sodium transport in the luminal membranes through eNaC channels

It causes reabsorption of Na and secretion of K^+ and H^+.
Acts on sweat, salivary and intestinal epithelium → retains Na^+ and Cl^- and loses K^+. As water is absorbed in the same concentration it does not change the concentration in the ECF.

Prostaglandins:

Produced from arachidonic acid when renal blood flow is compromised.
Prostacyclin (PGI2)- Afferent arteriole vasodilatation → ↑ RBF + GFR.

Atrial natriuretic peptide:

Released by special cells in the cardiac atria when they are stretched. Inhibits reabsorption of Na⁺ and water by the renal tubules, especially in the collecting ducts thus causing a natriuresis.

Thirst:

Thirst is stimulated by ↑ osmolarity, ↓ blood volume (e.g. haemorrhage), ↑ATII and a dry mouth. It is controlled by the hypothalamus.

ADH:

This allows for the kidney to excrete water independently of the rate of solute excretion so it *determines the osmolarity of the urine*.
Released from the posterior pituitary in response to increased plasma osmolarity. Osmoreceptors in the anterior hypothalamus; ↑ Osmolarity, ↓ cell size and nerve fibres signal to the posterior pituitary which causes the posterior pituitary to release ADH. Also stimulated by nausea, hypoxia, nicotine + morphine. Alcohol inhibits ADH hence causes a diuresis.

Action: In the late distal tubules, collecting tubules, and collecting ducts it binds to specific V2 receptors. This ↑ cyclic AMP and activating protein kinases to move aquaporin-2 (AQP-2) to the luminal side of the cell membranes. The molecules of AQP-2 cluster together and fuse with the cell membrane by exocytosis to form water channels that permit rapid diffusion of water through the cells.
ADH allows the body to conserve water; with maximum ADH secretion the urine osmolarity can ↑ to 1200 mOsm/L (4× plasma conc). Where as in states of water excess, water can be lost in excess of solutes and the urine osmolarity will be low; 50 mOsm/L.

Diuretics:
The definition of a diuretic is a substance that increases the rate of urine volume output. This is mainly through causing a natriuresis (Na⁺ loss), which subsequently causes a diuresis (water loss).

1. Osmotic diuretics-
   This is when there is high concentration of substances ('osmotic load') in the tubules that are not reabsorbed. e.g. Mannitol. Glucose can act as an osmotic diuretic when the concentration is higher than the transport maximum for glucose in the proximal tubule. Osmotic agents keep water in the tubular lumen.

2. Carbonic anhydrase inhibitor- e.g. Acetazolamide-
   Inhibits H⁺ secretion and therefore HCO₃⁻ reabsorption in the proximal tubules. This prevents the Na/H antiporter absorbing Na⁺, therefore overwhelming the distal tubules ability to absorb Na⁺.

3. Loop Diuretics- e.g. Frusemide-
   Inhibits the NaK2Cl channel in the thick ascending LoH. This delivers a higher solute load to the DCT, which causes an osmotic diuresis as well as disrupts the medullary interstitial osmolarity. As Na⁺ reabsorption is coupled to K⁺ secretion in the collecting duct, loop diuretics can lead to excessive K⁺ loss and hypokalemia.

4. Thiazide-
   Inhibits the NaCl transporter in the early DCT. As with loop diuretics, thiazide may also increase K+ loss and therefore may cause hypokalemia.

5. Aldosterone antagonist. e.g. Spironolactone-
   Inhibits that action of aldosterone in the DCT + collecting tubules.

5.5 Acid Base

Questions

1. How is HCO_3^- handled in the kidney (filtered, secreted or reabsorbed)
   HCO_3^- is freely filtered at the glomerulus and then reabsorbed along the collecting system (usually near 100% is reabsorbed).

2. Explain why the pH of the proximal tubules can not exceed pH 6.7, but in the distal collecting duct and collecting tubules the pH can get as low as 4.5.
   In the proximal tubules, the secretion of H^+ is via secondary active transport. Where as in the latter tubules the H^+ is actively secreted by the H^+ ATPase and this can pump against a high concentration gradient.

3. What is the most important urinary buffer?
   Phosphate is most important in the kidneys. This is for two reasons; (1) phosphate is poorly reabsorbed so concentration increases in the tubular lumen, thereby increasing the buffering (2) the pH in tubular fluid has a lower pH than blood, so it is closer to phosphate pKa of 6.8.

4. How is ammonia formed in the kidney?
   This is by the metabolism of glutamine. Glutamine is converted to 2× HCO_3^- and 2× NH_4^+. This NH_4^+ is secreted into the tubule and the HCO_3^- is free to diffuse into the blood stream.

Acid-base
The kidneys are very important for acid base balance. 80 milliequivalents of nonvolatile acid is produced by metabolism per day. This needs to be excreted in the kidney. The control of acid-base is a balance between the net loss and gain of H^+ and HCO_3^-.

- HCO_3^- is freely filtered in the glomerulus and then usually 100% reabsorbed. If excreted into the urine, this removes base from the blood.
- H^+ is not freely filtered but needs to be secreted.

Thus, the kidneys regulate extracellular fluid pH through three fundamental mechanisms: (1) secretion of H^+ (2) reabsorption of filtered HCO_3^- and (3) production of new HCO_3^-.
The titratable acidity is the amount of alkali that is added to urine to return the pH to 7.4 (the pH of the glomerular filtrate) (Fig. 5.9)
In the PCT, LoH and early DCT 80–90% of filtered HCO_3^- is reabsorbed.

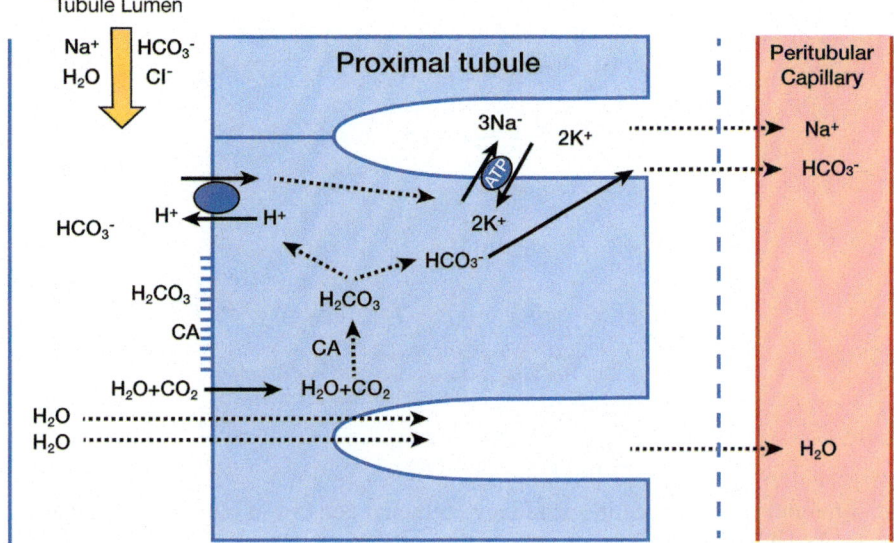

Fig. 5.9 Acid-base handling in the PCT

Firstly H⁺ is secreted via the NaH anti-porter, powdered by the basolateral Na/K ATPase.

Once inside the lumen, H⁺ and HCO_3^- then bind with the help of the luminal membrane carbonic anhydrase. This forms CO_2 and H_2O, the CO_2 can diffuse across into the cell. Once inside the cell, the CO_2 binds with H_2O (catalyzed by carbonic anhydrase) to produce H⁺ and HCO_3^-. The HCO_3^- then diffuses out of the basolateral aspect of the cell. In this way, the filtered HCO_3^- is effectively absorbed.

In the distal DCT and CT the last 10% is reabsorbed- Inside the cell, CO_2 and H_2O, with the help of carbonic anhydrase, combines to form H⁺ and HCO_3^-. The HCO_3^- diffuses out of the cell into the blood stream and the H⁺ is secreted into the lumen by H⁺ATPase.

This is only 5% of the total secreted H⁺ but it plays an important role in the acidification of urine. In the proximal tubules, the pH of the luminal fluid never exceeds 6.7 as the secretion is not through an active pump. In the latter part the pH can reach 4.5, as the secretion is active via the H+ ATPase (Fig. 5.10).

Tubular buffering

If there is excess H⁺ in the tubules after all HCO_3^- has been reabsorbed, it will combine with phosphates and ammonia.

Phosphate is the most important buffer in the kidney for two reasons: (1) phosphate is poorly reabsorbed so concentration increases in the tubular lumen, thereby increasing the buffering power of the phosphate system (2) the pH in tubular fluid has a lower pH so closer to phosphate pKa of 6.8,

Whenever tubular H⁺ combines with HPO_4^{2-} to form $H_2PO_4^-$ there is a net gain of HCO_3^- to the blood stream.

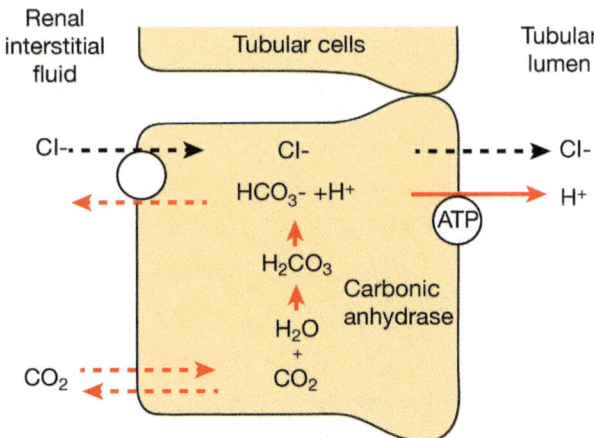

Fig. 5.10 Acid-base handling in the CT

Ammonia is produced in the kidney epithelial cells from glutamine (Glutamine → 2× HCO_3^- + 2× NH_4^+).

NH_4^+ is then secreted into the urine and the HCO_3^- is free to pass into the blood stream.

In situations of chronic acid base change, the kidney is stimulated to metabolise glutamine to produce new HCO_3^- and then secrete acid in the urine in the form of NH_4^+. This is the predominant mechanism in chronic acidosis.

5.6 Ion Transport

Questions

1. How is Na^+ absorbed from the proximal tubule?
   This is by secondary active transport. The Na/K ATPase on the basolateral membrane decreases the intracellular concentration of Na and allows for passive diffusion of luminal Na^+ down its concentration gradient. Many other substances are absorbed via co-transport with Na e.g. glucose and amino acids. 65% of filtered Na^+ is absorbed here.

2. How is Na^+ handled in the Loop of Henle?

   There are two channels in the ascending LoH. The NaK2Cl channel and the Na–H anti-porter.
   Remember that the descending limb of LoH is permeable to water, but relatively impermeable to ions.

3. How is HCO_3^- absorbed from the proximal tubule?
   This is via a rather convoluted pathway. H^+ is secreted into the tublular lumen via the Na/H^+ anti-porter in the PCT. The H^+ in the tubular lumen combines with the HCO_3^-, to form H_2O and CO_2. This CO_2 diffuses back into the cell, combines

5 Renal Physiology

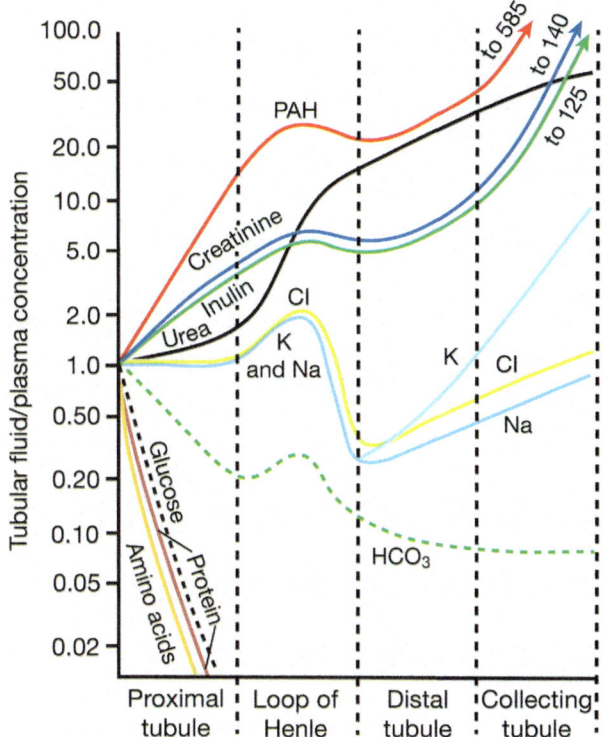

Fig. 5.11 Solute handling

with H_2O and then H^+ and HCO_3^- is formed. The HCO_3^- concentration increases and then HCO_3^- diffuses out of the basolateral aspect of the cell, leaving the H^+ to be secreted via the process described above.

4. How do principal cells handle Na?
   Principal cells absorb Na from the tubular lumen, under the control of Aldosterone. Basolateral Na/K ATPase maintains a low Na^+ concentration inside the cell and, therefore, favors Na^+ diffusion into the cell through special transport proteins.

5. What pH can the urine be concentrated to?
   pH 4.5. Can be secreted against a concentration gradient until a urine pH of approximately 4.5. This is achieved by the intercalated cells (Fig. 5.10).

Sodium:
Sodium absorption is important because it is closely linked with the reabsorption of water and it is the most numerous ECF ion.
PCT: 65% of filtered Na is reabsorbed here.
This is driven by the Na/K ATPase in the basolateral side (3Na out/2K in). This lowers intracellular Na^+ and sets up a concentration gradient for the facilitated diffusion of Na.

In the first half of PCT it is coupled to amino acid and glucose reabsorption, in the second half it is coupled with Cl reabsorption (Fig. 5.12).

LoH: About 25% of the filtered load of sodium is reabsorbed here.

This is in the ascending limb of LoH, once again powered by the basolateral Na/K ATPase, which drives the luminal transport of Na through the NaK2Cl.

There is also the Na-H anti-porter in the thick ascending LoH.

Early DCT: About 5% of the filtered load of sodium.

NaCl co-transporter moves sodium chloride from the tubular lumen into the cell, which then moves out the basolateral side due to the Na/K ATPase.

Late Distal Tubule and Collecting Tubule: Variable amount.

Principal cells- Na reabsorption and K secretion under the influence of Aldosterone. Basolateral Na/K ATPase maintains a low intracellular Na^+ concentration and, therefore, favors sodium diffusion into the cell through special transport proteins.

Chloride

PCT: 65% of Cl^- is reabsorbed here
Three mechanisms:

1. Anti-porter mechanism- Organic anions in exchange for Cl^-
2. Secondary active transport with Na^+
3. Na^+ and HCO_3^- ions are rapidly reabsorbed early in PCT, the concentration of Cl^- ions left in the tubular fluid rises, setting up a concentration gradient for paracellular diffusion of Cl^-

LoH: About 25% of the filtered load of Cl^-. This is in the ascending limb of LoH, via the NaK2Cl.

Early DCT: NaCl co-transporter moves sodium chloride from the tubular lumen into the cell, this is an example of secondary active transport.

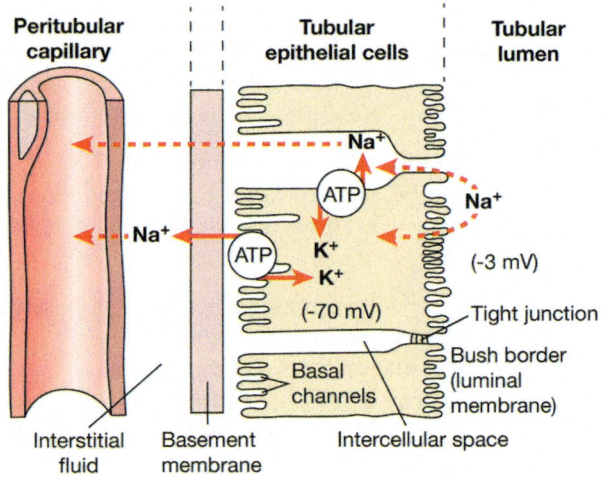

Fig. 5.12 Na^+ handling in the PCT

Potassium

This is largely an intracellular ion. It's ECF concentration is maintained closely. If there are large changes in ECF, can buffer it by shunting into the intracellular compartment.

Need to buffer against large changes in K^+ after a meal, therefore, insulin helps to shunt K^+ into the cell. Hyperkalaemia also stimulates Aldosterone secretion, which then increases the K loss in the kidney. Catecholamines, especially adrenaline can move K^+ into cells.

PT: 65% reabsorbed
LoH: 25–30% reabsorbed (NaK2Cl)

Distal Convoluted Tubule and Collecting Tubule: The amount of K^+ secreted and absorbed is altered in the in the DCT and CD.

With high K^+ concentration- large amount is secreted in DCT and CD.

With low K^+ concentration- K^+ can be reabsorbed. Always need to secrete 1% of filtered load, so if this is more than the daily intake then extreme hypokalaemia can ensue.

It is the principal cells of the DCT and CD that secrete K^+. This is through the action of the basolateral Na K ATPase, which causes an increased intracellular concentration of K^+; K^+ can diffuse down its concentration gradient, as the luminal membrane is permeable to K+.

Aldosterone increases the rate of secretion by increasing the Na K ATPase and also increasing the luminal permeability of K^+.

The K+ can be absorbed when there is whole body depletion and this is in the intercalated cells.

Increased GFR, increases K+ loss as it flushes away the K^+ in the lumen of the CD and sets up a concentration gradient for diffusion (Fig. 5.13).

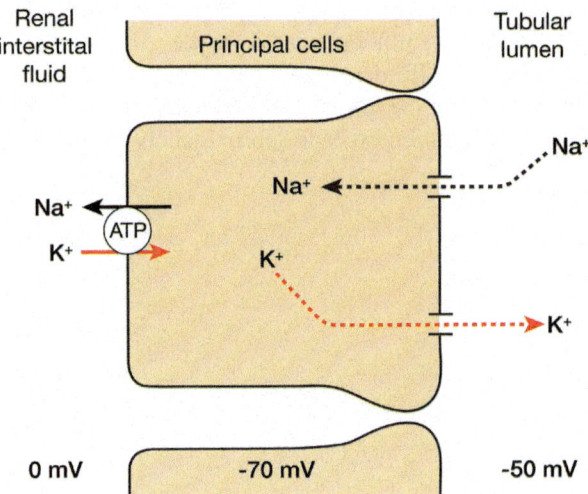

Fig. 5.13 K+ handling in principal cells

Water

To be able to excrete hyperosmolar urine need;

1. Anti-diuretic hormone (ADH)
2. High medullary interstitial osmolarity

PCT: Very permeable to water molecules. Water is thus reabsorbed by osmosis via both trans-cellular and para-cellular routes. Solutes and water are absorbed in the same amount, therefore there is little change in osmolarity.

LoH: The descending LoH is permeable to water so it moves down its concentration gradient. The tubular fluid is therefore hypertonic by the time the tubular fluid reaches the end of the descending LoH. The ascending LoH is not permeable to water. The luminal fluid is therefore hypotonic by the time it reaches the DCT.

Descending LoH- water absorption in excess of solute = hyperosmotic
Ascending LoH- solute absorption in excess of water = hypoosmotic

Early DCT: Virtually impermeable to water

Late Distal Tubule, Collecting Tubule and Duct: Under control of ADH. In the absence of ADH there is no water absorption. In the presence of ADH there is maximal absorption.

Glucose

Glucose is fully filtered at the glomerulus.

PCT: Normally, 100% of filtered glucose is reabsorbed in the PCT.

This is by secondary active transport with sodium glucose co-transporter type 2 (SGLT-2). The SGLT-2 in the apical membrane binds the glucose and the Na^+. When the Na^+ moves down the electrochemical gradient, glucose moves into the cell as well. Glucose then moves out of the cell via the glucose transporter 2 (GLUT2) on the basolateral aspect.

This process can be saturated. The rate at which this occurs is called the tubular maximum, T_{max}. When the filtered load of glucose exceeds T_{max} glucose will be present in the filtrate after the proximal tubule. This will create an osmotic gradient thus retaining water in the filtrate and increasing diuresis. This happens if the plasma glucose concentration exceeds approximately 10 mmol/L.

Index

A
Acetylcholine (Ach), 2, 9, 27, 38, 42, 44, 61, 69, 80, 98, 127
Acid dissociation constant (pKa), 132, 133
Adrenocorticotropic hormone (ACTH), 2, 3, 5, 6, 11–14, 73, 75, 130
Alveolar partial pressure (PA), 93, 95
Alveolar partial pressure (Pa), 93, 95
Ammonium (NH_4^+), 132, 134
Angiotensin converting enzyme (ACE), 11, 74, 130
Angiotensin II (ATII), 2–4, 11, 12, 71, 72, 74, 75, 78, 98, 100, 127, 129–131
Anterior pituitary (AP), 3–6, 13, 15, 16, 18, 31, 32, 34–36, 130
Anti-diuretic hormone (ADH), 3–5, 23, 52, 71, 73, 75, 78, 123, 129–131, 138
Aquaporin-2 (AQP-2), 129–131
Area (A), 37, 42, 45, 53, 83, 84, 87, 89, 92–95, 99, 121, 127
Arterial concentration (Ca), 67, 125
Arterial concentration of oxygen (CaO_2), 67, 97
Arterial partial pressure (Pa), 104
Atrial fibrillation (AF), 19, 66
Atrial natriuretic peptide (ANP), 2, 73, 75, 131
Atrioventricular (AV), 55–58, 60, 61, 63, 64, 66, 67, 69, 80, 84
Autonomic nervous system (ANS), 69, 73

B
Barometric Pressure (P_B), 102
Basal metabolic rate (BMR), 19, 35
Basic electrical rhythm (BER), 38, 129

Bicarbonate (HCO3-), 47, 51, 104, 106
Blood flow (BF), 38, 39, 68, 70, 73, 74, 76, 77, 80–85, 95–97, 99, 102, 103, 114, 123–125, 127, 130
Blood pressure (BP), 12, 71–75, 80, 84, 88, 97–99, 115
Blood vessels (BV), 3, 5, 70, 71, 75, 130

C
Calcium (Ca^{2+}), 2, 3, 5, 9, 19–26, 31, 38, 39, 41, 47, 61, 63, 64, 68, 69, 77, 107, 124, 127
Capillary partial pressure (Pc), 96, 99, 127
Carbon dioxide (CO_2), 77, 100, 104, 106, 115
Carbon Monoxide (CO), 93, 95
Cardiac output (CO), 67–68, 76, 83, 86, 96, 97
Cardiac output (Q), 67, 68, 76, 83, 86, 96, 97
Cardiovascular system (CVS), 18, 72–74
Catechol-O-methyltransferases (COMT), 9
Central nervous sytem (CNS), 18–20, 41
Cerebral perfusion pressure (CPP), 77, 80
Cerebrospinal fluid (CSF), 77, 80, 113, 114
Chloride (Cl-), 2, 39, 41, 42, 46, 51, 75, 107, 118–124, 127, 130, 131, 134, 136, 137
Cholecystokinin (CCK), 4, 25, 27, 29, 39, 42, 46, 47
Chronic renal failure (CRF), 24
Collecting ducts (CD), 3, 4, 72, 75, 121–123, 129–132, 137
Collecting tubules (CT), 121, 123, 129, 131, 132, 136–138
Corticosteroid-binding globulin (CBG), 11, 14
Corticotropin-releasing hormone (CRH), 6, 13

Cranial nerve (CN), 113
Cyclic AMP (cAMP), 2, 4, 9, 13, 22, 27, 64, 69, 131
Cyclooxygenase (COX), 78

D

Dehydroepiandrosterone (DHEA), 14, 34
Density (p), 82, 85, 109–111
Deoxyribonucleic acid (DNA), 2, 18, 23, 51
Diffusion capacity of the lung (DL), 93, 95
Diffusion coefficient (D), 94
1,25-dihydroxycholecalciferol (1,25 DHCC), 19, 22, 23
2,3-Diphosphoglyceric acid (DPG), 106
Distal convoluted tubule (DCT), 121, 123–125, 127, 130–133, 136–138

E

Ejection fraction (EF), 56, 60, 70, 76
End diastolic volume (EDV), 55, 56, 58–60, 67, 70, 71, 76
Endoplasmic reticulum (ER), 2, 21
Endothelium-derived relaxing factor (EDRF), 77, 78
End systolic volume (ESV), 55, 58, 60
Enteric nervous system (ENS), 38, 39
Enterochromaffin-like (ECL), 42, 44, 46, 47
Epidermal growth factor (EGF), 2, 7
Erythropoietin (EPO), 72, 75
Estimated glomerular filtration rate (eGFR), 125, 127
Expiratory reserve volume (ERV), 90, 91
Extracellular fluid (ECF), 11, 13–16, 19–21, 35, 73, 75, 113, 114, 117–120, 129, 130, 132, 135, 137

F

Fetal haemoglobin (HbF), 30, 33
Follicle stimulating hormone (FSH), 5–7, 29, 31, 32, 34, 36
Fraction of inspired oxygen (FiO2), 100
Free fatty acid (FFA), 28
Functional Residual Capacity (FRC), 90, 91, 96, 108, 110, 111

G

Gallbladder (GB), 41, 46, 47
Gamma-Aminobutyric acid (GABA), 2, 27
G-Protein coupled receptor (GPCR), 23

Gastric inhibitory polypeptide (GIP), 27, 48
Gastrin releasing peptide (GRP), 44
Gastrointestinal tract (GIT), 18, 19, 37, 40, 41
Glomerular ultra filtration coefficient (kf), 125, 127
Glucose transporter 2 (GLUT2), 48, 49, 138
Gonadotropin-releasing hormone (GnRH), 6, 31, 36
Growth hormone (GH), 2, 5–7, 23, 28, 29, 35
Growth hormone–inhibiting hormone (GHIH), 6, 7
Growth hormone releasing hormone (GHRH), 6, 7

H

Haemoglobin (Hb), 30, 33, 41, 51, 93, 95, 103–106
Heart rate (HR), 18, 57, 61, 65, 69, 74, 76
Heart sound (HS), 58
Human chorionic gonadotropin (hCG), 33
Hydrochloric acid (HCl), 11, 14, 42–44, 46, 47, 49, 53
Hydrogen (H^+), 12, 51, 78, 81, 106, 113, 114, 121–123, 129–135
Hydrogen ATPase transporter (H^+ ATPase), 121, 123, 132, 133

I

Inferior vena cava (IVC), 77, 82
Inspiratory capacity (IC), 91
Inspiratory reserve volume (IRV), 90, 91
Insulin-like growth factor 1 (IGF-I), 7
Intracellular fluid (ICP), 77, 80
Intracranial pressure (ICP), 77, 80
Intrinsic factor (IF), 42, 43, 51–53
Iodide (I^-), 15–17

J

Jugular venous pressure (JVP), 56, 58, 59
Juxtaglomerular (JG), 11, 72–74, 129

L

Large intestine (LI), 42–46, 54
Left atrium (LA), 65, 82
Left ventricle (LV), 60, 73, 80, 83, 101, 102
Length (l), 61, 67, 68, 82, 84, 109, 111
Linear dimention (L), 111
Litre (L), 4, 20, 21, 23, 26, 39, 42, 46, 72, 76, 83, 117, 119, 121, 129, 131, 138

Litre per day (L/day), 4, 117, 118, 121, 122, 127
Loop of Henle (LI), 21, 121–125, 134
Lower esophageal sphincter (LES), 52
Luteinizing hormone (LH), 5–7, 9, 31, 32, 34–36

M

Magnesium (Mg^{2+}), 51
Mean arterial blood pressure (MABP), 71, 73, 74, 84, 125
Mean hydrostatic pressure in the glomerular capillaries (P_{GC}), 125, 127
Mean hydrostatic pressure in the tubule (Bowman's space) (P_T), 125, 128
Melanocyte-stimulating hormones (MSH), 11, 14
Millilittres per minute (mL/min), 67, 73, 76, 77, 88, 121, 125, 127
Mineralocorticoid receptor (MR), 12, 130
Molecular weight (MW), 78, 93, 94, 129
Monoamine oxidases (MAO), 9, 10
Multiple organ dysfunction sundrome (MODS), 72
Musculoskeletal system (MSK), 18

N

Nerve growth factor (NGF), 7
Net filtration pressure (P_{UF}), 129
Nitric oxide (NO), 76, 96
Nitrous oxide (N_2O), 93, 95
Noradrenaline (NA), 8–10, 73, 74, 81, 123, 127, 130
Nucleus tractus solitarius (NTS), 74

O

Oncotic pressure in the filtrate of the tubule (πT), 125, 129

P

Para-aminohippuric acid (PAH), 123, 125
Parasympathetic nervous system (PSNS), 61, 68, 69, 74, 78, 79
Parathyroid hormone (PTH), 2, 18–24
Parathyroid hormone-related protein (PTHrP), 24
Partial pressure (P), 93–95, 99, 101, 104–106
Phenylethanolamine-N-methyltransferase (PNMT), 8

Phosphate (PO_4^{-3}), 19–21, 24, 51, 118, 132, 133
Phospholipase C (PLC), 2, 9
Platelet-derived growth factor (PDGF), 2, 7
Potassium (K^+), 51, 118, 137
Pro-opiomelanocortin (POMC), 11, 14
Prostacyclin (PGI2), 78, 127, 130
Proximal convoluted tubule (PCT), 122, 132–136, 138
Pulmonary embolism (PE), 71, 109

R

Radius (r), 82–85, 109, 111
Rate of gas transfer (V), 94
Rate of O_2 consumption (VO2), 97
Red blood cell (RBC), 26, 27, 35, 51–53, 74, 75, 90, 95, 106, 107
Renal blood flow (RBF), 123–130
Renin-Angiotensin-Aldosterone system (RAAS), 70, 74
Residual Volume (RV), 82, 90, 91
Respiratory rate (RR), 18, 65
Resting membrane potential (RMP), 61, 63, 64
Right atrium (RA), 58, 61, 82, 97, 99

S

Saturation (S), 95, 105
Sinoatrial (SA), 61, 64, 69
Smooth muscle (SM), 3, 5, 10, 27, 38, 48, 73, 88, 98, 112, 115
Sodium (Na^+), 12, 13, 18, 19, 50, 51, 74, 118, 119, 126, 130, 135, 136, 138
Sodium/Chloride transporter (NaCl), 13, 121, 123, 132, 136
Sodium glucose co-transporter type 2 (SGLT-2), 138
Sodium/Potassium ATPase transporter (Na/K ATPase), 62, 121–124, 127, 130, 133–136
Sodium/Potassium/2xChloride transporter (NAK2Cl), 121, 122, 124, 127, 130, 131, 134, 136, 137
Stroke volume (SV), 55, 60, 67, 68, 71
Sympathetic nervous system (SNS), 64, 70, 73, 74, 130
Systolic blood pressure (SBP), 9, 10, 84, 98

T

Terminal ileum (TI), 40, 49
Testis determining factor (TDF), 34
Thickness (T), 35, 83, 92–95

Thromboxane A2 (TXA2), 76, 78
Thyroid releasing hormone
(TRH), 2, 6, 15, 16
Thyroid stimulating hormone (TSH), 2, 5, 6,
15–17, 19
Thyroxine-binding globulin (TBG), 18
Tidal volume (TV), 90, 91
Total body calcium (TBC), 20
Total Lung Capacity (TLC), 91
Total peripheral resistance (TPR), 71–73, 75
Toxic multinodular goiter (TMNG), 19
Transcortin (CBG), 11, 14
Triglycerides (TGs), 18, 25, 27, 48–50, 125
Tubuloglomerular feedback
(TGF), 74, 123–125

V
Vasoactive intestinal polypeptide
(VIP), 39, 48, 80
Velocity (u), 82, 85, 109, 111
Venous concentration of oxygen (CvO2), 67
Ventilation/Perfusion (V/Q), 100, 102, 103
Ventricular fibrillation (VF), 66
Viscosity (μ), 80, 82, 84, 85, 109, 111
Vital Capacity (VC), 91, 111

W
Water (H2O), 40, 45, 51, 80, 87, 99, 106,
117–124, 129–131, 133–135, 138
Wolf-Parkinson-White (WPW), 67

The manufacturer's authorised representative in the EU is Springer Nature Customer Service Centre GmbH, Europaplatz 3, 69115 Heidelberg, Germany. If you have any concerns regarding our products, please contact ProductSafety@springernature.com

Printed and bound by CPI Group (UK) Ltd, Croydon, CR0 4YY

25/03/2026

02078176-0003